The Lost Art of Listening

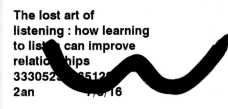
The Lost Art
of Listening

• • •

How Learning to Listen
Can Improve Relationships

SECOND EDITION

Michael P. Nichols

THE GUILFORD PRESS
New York   London

Published by The Guilford Press
A Division of Guilford Publications, Inc.
370 Seventh Avenue, Suite 1200, New York, NY 10001
www.guilford.com

Printed in the United States of America

This book is printed on acid-free paper.

Last digit is print number: 9   8   7   6   5

Library of Congress Cataloging-in-Publication Data

Nichols, Michael P.
    The lost art of listening : how learning to listen can improve relationships / Michael P. Nichols. — 2nd. ed.
        p.   cm.
    Includes index.
    ISBN 978-1-60623-064-0 (hardcover : alk. paper)
    ISBN 978-1-59385-986-2 (pbk. : alk. paper)
    1. Listening.   2. Interpersonal relations.   3. Interpersonal communication.   I. Title.
    BF323.L5N53 2009
    153.6′8—dc22
                                         2008054617

Contents

Part Three
• • •
Getting Through to Each Other

Part Four
• • •
Listening in Context

Introduction

Nothing hurts more than the sense that the people we care about aren't really listening. We never outgrow the need to have our feelings known. That's why a sympathetic ear is such a powerful force in human relationships—and why the failure to be understood is so painful.

My ideas about listening have been sharpened by thirty-five years as a psychoanalyst and family therapist. Refereeing arguments between intimate partners, coaching parents to communicate with their children, and struggling myself to sustain empathy as my patients faced their demons has led me to the conclusion that much of the conflict in our lives can be explained by one simple fact: people don't really listen to each other.

Talking without listening is like snipping an electrical cord in half and hoping that somehow something will light up. Most of the time, of course, we don't deliberately set out to break the connection. In fact, we're often baffled and dismayed by feeling left in the dark.

Modern culture has developed conceptions of individualism that picture us finding our own bearings within, declaring independence from the webs of interlocution that formed us. It's as though when we become finished persons we outgrow our need for attention, like training wheels. All this is not to say that we can't be autonomous, in the sense of being self-directing, even original, able to think and act on our own. But we cannot escape the human condition and become secure and satisfied without conversation—conversation in a broad sense, meaning some kind of interchange with others.

1

Contemporary pressures have, regrettably, shrunk our attention spans and impoverished the quality of listening in our lives. We live in hurried times, when dinner is something you zap in the microwave and keeping up with the latest books and movies means reading the reviews. That's all we've got time for. Running to and from our many obligations, we get a lot of practice in not listening. When we're in the car and the radio is on, sometimes it's interesting and we pay attention, other times we have to concentrate on the road or we get sidetracked with a thought, and minutes go by without our hearing a word of what was said. When we're watching TV and the commercials come on, half the time we don't hear a thing.

We're bombarded with so many images—from television, e-mail, junk mail, the Internet, cell phones, BlackBerrys, iPods, pagers, faxes—that our attention is fractionated. We like to think we're good at multitasking. We check our e-mail while talking on the phone. We look for things to buy in catalogues while watching TV. We fool ourselves into thinking that we can do more than one thing at a time. The truth is that we just end up doing one thing after another poorly.

We've gained unparalleled access to information and lost something very important. We've lost the habit of concentrating our attention. From pop music at the gym to commercials on TV and radio, we're bombarded with so much noise that we've become experts at tuning things out. If a television show doesn't grab our attention in the first two minutes, we change the channel; if we're listening to someone who doesn't get right to something we're interested in, we tune out.

In the limited time we still preserve for family and friends, conversation is often preempted by soothing and passive distractions. Too tired to talk and listen, we settle instead for the lulling charms of electronic devices that project pictures, make music, or bleep across display screens. Is it this way of life that's made us forget how to listen? Perhaps. But maybe the modern approach to life is the effect rather than the cause of the decline of meaningful discourse. Maybe we lead this kind of life because we're seeking some sort of solace, something to counteract the dimming of the spirit we feel when no one is listening.

How we lost the art of listening is certainly a matter for debate. What isn't debatable is that the loss leaves us with an ever-widening hole in our lives. It might take the form of a vague sense of discontent, sadness, or deprivation. We miss the consolation of lending an attentive ear and of receiving the same in return, but we don't know what's wrong or how to fix it. Over time this lack of listening impoverishes our most important relationships. We hurt each other unnecessarily by failing to acknowledge what the other one has to say. Whatever the arena, our hearts experience the failure to be heard as an absence of concern.

Conflict doesn't necessarily disappear when we acknowledge each other's point of view, but it's almost certain to get worse if we don't. So why don't we take time to hear each other? Because the simple art of listening isn't so simple.

Often it's a burden. Not, perhaps, the perfunctory attention we grant as part of the give-and-take of everyday life. But the sustained attention of careful listening—that takes strenuous and unselfish restraint. To listen well we must forget ourselves and submit to the other person's need for attention.

While some people may be easier to listen to than others, conversations take place between two people, both of whom contribute to the outcome. Unfortunately, when we fail to get through to each other, we have a tendency to fall back on blaming. It's his fault: he's selfish and insensitive. Or it's my fault: I'm too dependent or don't express myself well.

Most failures of understanding are not due to self-absorption or bad faith, but to our own need to say something. We tend to react to what is said, rather than concentrating on what the other person is trying to express. Emotional reactions make us respond without thinking and crowd out understanding and concern. Each of us has characteristic ways of reacting defensively. We don't hear what's said because something in the speaker's message triggers hurt, anger, or impatience.

Unfortunately, all the advice in the world about "active listening" can't overcome the maddening tendency to react defensively to each other. To become better listeners, and to transform our relationships, we must identify and harness the emotional triggers that generate anxiety and cause misunderstanding and conflict.

If this seems too formidable a task, remember that most of us are more capable than we give ourselves credit for. We concentrate pretty hard at work, and most of us still enjoy earnest, open conversation with a few friends. In fact, talking with friends is a model of what conversation can be: safe enough to talk about what matters, concerned enough to listen, honest enough to tell the truth, and tactful enough to know when not to. More relationships can be like this.

In the process of writing this book, I've tried to become a better listener, in my personal as well as professional life, to listen a little harder to my wife's complaints without getting defensive and to hear my children's opinions before giving my own. However, I've had a few conversations that left me feeling bruised and defeated. My wife would speak sharply to me about not helping out more around the house or not listening to her, and I'd feel attacked; or I'd call my editor one too many times to complain about the burdens of writing and she'd make *me* feel like a burden for complaining; or my friend Rich would call me the part of your anatomy you sit on for acting like I was entitled to some special consideration. Not only didn't I listen at these times—hear and acknowledge what the other person was saying—but I got hurt and angry, and completely unwilling to talk to that person, *ever again, as long as I live.*

I'm sure you know how painful such misunderstandings can be. When my wife "yelled at me," my editor was "mean to me," and my friend "picked on me," I got hurt and withdrew. But what made these incidents especially painful was that just when I thought I was learning to listen better, these setbacks set me all the way back. Instead of just thinking that things hadn't gone well and needed repair, I felt defeated and inadequate. How could I, who couldn't even get along with the people in my own life, have the temerity to write a book about listening? How could I teach anyone anything about communicating?

Maybe you know how that feels. When we try to change something in our lives, whether it's our diet or work habits or listening skills, and we experience a setback, we have a tendency to feel hopeless and give up. Suddenly all the progress we thought we were making seems like an illusion. Maybe if I were reading a book about listening and experienced these setbacks, I would have given up. But since I was *writing* this book, after a while of brooding in hurt silence I'd go back and try to talk to the person I'd quarreled with—only this time with a firm resolve to listen to his or her side before telling mine. In the process, I learned to see how my relationships go through cycles of closeness and distance and, even more important, how I could influence those cycles by the quality of my own listening.

This book is an invitation to think about the ways we talk and listen to each other: why listening is such a powerful force in our lives; how to listen deeply, with sustained immersion in another's experience; and how to prevent good listening from being spoiled by bad habits. Among the secrets of successful communication I'll describe are:

- The difference between real dialogue and just taking turns talking
- Hearing what people mean, not just what they say
- How to get through to someone who never seems to listen
- How to reduce arguments
- How to ask for support without getting unwanted advice
- How to get uncommunicative people to open up
- How to share a difference of opinion without making other people feel criticized
- How to make sure both sides get heard in heated discussions
- How speakers undermine their own messages
- How the nature of relationships affects listening
- How to get people to listen to you

The Lost Art of Listening is divided into four sections. Part I explains why listening is so important in our lives—far more important than we realize—and how, for many people, it's a lack of sympathetic attention, not stress or overwork, that accounts for the loss of enthusiasm and optimism in their lives. Part II explores the hidden assumptions, unconscious needs, and emotional reactions that are the real reasons people don't listen. We'll see what makes listeners too defensive to hear what others are saying and why you may not get heard even though you have something important to say.

After exploring the major roadblocks to listening, I'll examine in Part III how you can understand and control emotional reactivity to become a better listener. And I'll explain how you can make yourself heard, even in the most difficult situations. Finally, in Part IV, I'll explore how listening breaks down in particular types of relationship, including intimate partnerships, family relationships, with children, between friends, and at work. I'll explain how listening is complicated by the dynamics of each of these various relationships and how to use that knowledge to break through to each other.

At the end of each chapter, you'll find a set of exercises designed to help you become a better listener. Actually doing these exercises may help transform the passive experience of reading into an active process of improving your ability to listen.

Regardless of how much we take it for granted, the importance of listening cannot be overestimated. The gift of our attention and understanding makes other people feel validated and valued. Our ability to listen, and listen well, creates goodwill that comes back to us. But effective listening is also the best way to enjoy others, to learn from them, and to make them interesting to be with. I hope this book can help take us a step in the direction of showing more of the concern we feel for each other.

Part One

. . .

The Yearning
to Be Understood

1

• • •

"Did You Hear What I Said?"

Why Listening Is So Important

Sometimes it seems that nobody listens anymore.

> "He expects me to listen to his problems, but he never asks about mine."

> "She's always complaining."

> "The only time I find out what's going on in his life is when I overhear him telling someone else. Why doesn't he tell *me* these things?"

> "I can't talk to her because she's so critical."

Wives complain that their husbands take them for granted. Husbands complain that their wives nag or take forever to get to the point.

She feels a violation of their connection. He doesn't trust the connection.

Few motives in human experience are as powerful as the yearning to be understood. Being listened to means that we are taken seriously, that our ideas and feelings are recognized, and, ultimately, that what we have to say matters.

The yearning to be heard is a yearning to escape our isolation and bridge the space that separates us. We reach out and try to overcome that separateness by revealing what's on our minds and in our hearts, hoping for understanding. Getting that understanding should be simple, but it isn't.

Joan had seen a suit she'd like to buy for work, but wasn't sure she should spend the money. "Honey," she said, "I saw a really nice suit at the outlet store."

"That's nice," Henry said, and went back to watching the news.

Justin was upset about having had a fender bender, but he was afraid that if he said anything Denise would get on his case about it. So he kept quiet and worried about how he was going to get it fixed. Denise felt Justin's distance and assumed that he was angry at her for something. She didn't feel like having an argument, so she didn't say anything either.

The essence of good listening is empathy, which can be achieved only by suspending our preoccupation with ourselves and entering into the experience of the other person. Part intuition and part effort, it's the stuff of human connection.

A listener's empathy—grasping what we're trying to say *and showing it*—builds a bond of understanding, linking us to someone who hears us and cares, and thus confirms that our feelings are legitimate and recognizable. The power of empathic listening is the power to transform relationships. When deeply felt but unexpressed feelings take shape in words that are voiced and come back clarified, the result is a reassuring sense of being understood and a grateful feeling of shared humanness with the one who understands.

● ● ●

The art of listening is critical to successful relationships.

● ● ●

If listening strengthens our relationships by cementing our connection with one another, it also fortifies our sense of self. In the presence of a receptive listener, we are able to clarify what we think and discover what we feel. Thus, in giving an account of our experience to someone who listens, we are better able to listen to ourselves. Our lives are defined in dialogue.

It Hurts Not to Be Listened To

The need to be taken seriously and responded to is frustrated every day. Parents complain that their children don't listen. Children complain that their parents are too busy scolding to hear their side of things. Even friends, usually a reliable source of shared understanding, are often too busy to listen to one another these days. And if we sometimes feel cut off from sympathy and understanding in the private sphere, we've grown not even to expect courtesy and attention in public settings.

Our right to be heard is violated in countless ways that we don't always remember, by others who don't always realize. That doesn't make it hurt any less.

When I told a psychiatrist friend that I was collecting experiences on the theme "It hurts not to be listened to," he sent me this example:

"I called a friend and left a message asking if we could meet at a particular time. He didn't answer, and I felt a little anxious and confused. Should I call again to remind him? After all, I know he's busy. Should I wait another day or two and hope he'll answer? Should I not have asked him in the first place? All this leaves me uneasy."

The first thing that struck me about this example was how even a little thing like an unanswered phone message can leave someone feeling unresponded to—and troubled. Then I was really struck—like a slap in the face—by the realization that my friend was talking about me! Suddenly I was embarrassed, and then defensive. The reason I hadn't returned his call—doesn't matter. (We always have reasons for not responding.) What matters is how my failure to respond hurt and confused my friend and that I never had any inkling of it.

If an oversight like that can hurt, how much more painful is it when the subject is of urgent importance to the speaker?

• • •

Listening is so basic that we take it for granted. Unfortunately, most of us think of ourselves as better listeners than we really are.

• • •

When you come home from a business trip, eager to tell your partner how it went, and he listens but after a minute or two something in his eyes goes to sleep, you feel hurt and betrayed. When you call your parents to share a triumph and they don't seem really interested, you feel deflated and perhaps slightly foolish for having allowed yourself to even hope for appreciation.

Just as it hurts not to be listened to when you're excited about something special, it's painful not to feel listened to by someone special, someone you expect to care about you.

Roger's best friend in college was Derek. They were both political science majors and shared a passion for politics. Together they followed every detail of the Watergate investigation, relishing each new revelation as though they were a series of deliciously wicked Charles Addams cartoons. But as much as they took cynical delight in the exposure of corruption in the Nixon White House, their friendship went beyond politics.

Roger remembered the wonderful feeling of talking to Derek for hours, impelled by the momentum of some deep and inexplicable sympathy. There was the pleasure of being able to say anything he wanted and the pleasure of hearing Derek say everything he'd always thought but never expressed. Unlike most of Roger's other friends, Derek wasn't a competitive conversationalist. He really listened.

When they went to graduate schools in different cities, they kept up their friendship. Roger would visit Derek, or Derek would visit Roger, at least once a month. They'd play pool or see a movie and go out for Chinese food; and then afterward, no matter how late it got, they'd stay up talking.

Then Derek got married, and things changed. Derek didn't become distant the way some friends do after one marries, nor did Derek's wife dislike Roger. The distance that Roger felt was a small thing, but it made a big difference.

"It's difficult to describe exactly, but I often end up feeling awkward and disappointed when I speak with Derek. He listens, but somehow he doesn't seem really interested anymore. He doesn't ask questions. He used to be involved rather than just accepting. It makes me sad. I still feel excited about the things going on in my life, but telling Derek just makes me feel unconnected and alone with them."

Roger's lament says something important about listening. It isn't just not being interrupted that we want. Sometimes people appear to be listening but aren't really hearing. Some people are good at being silent when we talk. Sometimes they betray their lack of interest by glancing around and shifting their weight back and forth. At other times, however, listeners show no sign of inattention, but still we know they aren't really hearing what we have to say. It feels like they don't care.

Derek's passive interest was especially painful to Roger because of the closeness they'd shared. The friends had reached an impasse; Roger couldn't open himself to his friend the way he'd done in the past, and Derek was mystified by the distance that had grown between them.

Friendship is voluntary, and so talking about it is optional. Roger didn't want to complain to Derek or make demands. Besides, how does one friend tell another that he feels no longer cared about? And so Roger never did talk to Derek about feeling estranged. Too bad, because when a relationship goes sour, talking about it may be the only way to make things right again.

● ● ●

It's especially hurtful not to be listened to in those relationships we count on for understanding.

● ● ●

After a while most of us learn to do a pretty good imitation of being grownups and shrug off a lot of slights and misunderstandings. If, in the process, we become a little calloused, well maybe that's the price we pay for getting along in the world. But sometimes not being responded to leaves us feeling so hurt and angry that it can make us retreat from relationships, even for years.

When a woman discovered that her husband was having an affair, she felt as if someone had kicked her in the gut. In her grief and anger, she turned to the person she was closest to—her mother-in-law. The mother-in-law tried to be understanding and supportive, but it was, after all, difficult to listen to the bitter things her daughter-in-law was saying about her son. Still, she tried. Apparently, however, the support she offered wasn't enough. Eventually the crisis passed and the couple reconciled, but the daughter-in-law, feeling that her mother-in-law hadn't been there when she needed her most, never spoke to her again.

The mother-in-law in this sad story was baffled by her daughter-in-law's stubborn silence. Other people's reactions often seem unreasonable to us. What makes their reactions reasonable to them is feeling wounded by a lack of responsiveness.

To listen is to pay attention, take an interest, care about, take to heart, validate, acknowledge, be moved ... appreciate. Listening is so central to human existence as to often escape notice; or, rather, it appears in so many guises that it's seldom recognized as the overarching need that it is. Sometimes, as Roger, the estranged daughter-in-law, and so many others have discovered, we don't realize how important being listened to is until we feel cheated out of it.

Once in a while, however, we become aware of how much it means to be listened to. You can't decide whether or not to take a new job, and so you call an old friend to talk it over. She doesn't tell you what to do, but the fact that she listens, really listens, helps you see things more clearly. Another time you're just getting to know someone but you like him so much that, after a wonderful dinner in a restaurant, you take a risk and ask him over for coffee. When he says, "No thanks, I've got to get up early," you feel rejected. Convinced that he doesn't like you, you start avoiding him. After a few days, however, he asks you what's wrong, and once again you take a risk and tell him that your feelings were hurt. To your great relief, instead of arguing, he listens and accepts what you have to say. "I can see how you might have felt that way, but actually I would like to see you again."

Why can't it always be that way? I speak, you listen. It's that simple, isn't it? Unfortunately, it isn't. Talking and listening creates a unique relationship in which speaker and listener are constantly switching roles, both jockeying for position, each one's needs competing with the other's. If you doubt it, try telling someone about a problem you're having and see how long it takes before he interrupts to describe a similar experience of his own or to offer advice—advice that may suit him more than it does you.

A man in therapy was exploring his relationship with his distant father when he suddenly remembered the happy times they'd spent together playing with his electric trains. It was a Lionel set that had been his father's and grandfather's before him. Caught up in the memory, the man grew increasingly excited as he recalled the pride he'd felt in sharing this family tradition with his father. As the man's enthusiasm mounted, the therapist launched into a long narrative about *his* train set and how he had gotten the other kids in the neighborhood to bring over their tracks and train cars to build a huge neighborhood setup in his basement. After the therapist had gone on at some length, the patient could no longer contain his anger about being cut off. "Why are you telling me about *your* trains?!" he demanded. The therapist hesitated; then, with that level, impersonal voice we reserve for confiding something intimate, he said lamely, "I was just trying to be friendly."

● ● ●

It takes two people to share a feeling—one to talk and one to listen.

● ● ●

The therapist had made an all-too-common mistake (actually he'd made several, but this is Be Kind to Therapists Week). He assumed that sharing his own experience was the equivalent of empathy. In fact, though, he switched the focus to himself, making his patient feel discounted, misunderstood, unappreciated. That's what hurt.

As is often the way with words that become familiar, *empathy* may not adequately convey the power of appreciating the inner experience of another person. Empathic listening is like the close reading of a poem; it takes in the words and gets to what's behind them. The difference is that while empathy is actively imaginative, it is fundamentally receptive rather than creative. When we attend to a work of art, our idiosyncratic response has its own validity, but when we attend to someone who's trying to tell us something, it's understanding, not creativity, that counts.

Bearing Witness

Listening has not one but two purposes: taking in information and bearing witness to another's experience. By momentarily stepping out of his or her own frame of reference and into ours, the person who really listens acknowledges and affirms us. That validation is essential for sustaining the confirmation known as self-respect. Without being listened to, we are shut up in the solitude of our own hearts.

A thirty-six-year-old woman was so unnerved by a minor incident that she wondered if she needed psychotherapy. Marnie, who was executive vice-president of a public policy institute, had arranged a meeting with the lieutenant governor to present a proposal she'd developed involving the regulation of a large state industry. Of necessity she'd invited her boss to the meeting, although she would have been able to make a more effective presentation without him. The boss, in turn, had invited the institute's chief lobbyist, who would later have to convince legislators of the need for the proposed regulation. The meeting began, as Marnie expected, with her boss rambling on in a loose philosophical discussion that circled but never quite got to the point. When he finished, he turned not to Marnie but to the lobbyist to present the proposal. Marnie was stunned. The lobbyist began to speak, and fifteen minutes later the meeting ended without Marnie's ever having gotten to say a word—about *her* proposal.

Marnie couldn't wait to tell her husband what had happened. Unfortunately he was in Europe and wouldn't be back for three days. She was used to her husband's business trips; what she wasn't used to was how cut off she felt. She really needed to talk to him. As the evening wore on, Marnie's disappointment grew and then changed character. Instead of simply feeling frustrated, she began to feel inadequate. Why was she so dependent on her husband? Why couldn't she handle her own emotions?

Marnie decided that her problem was insecurity. If she were more secure, she wouldn't need anyone so much. She wouldn't be so vulnerable; she'd be self-sufficient.

Marnie's complaint—the unexpected urgency to be heard—and her conclusion, that if she'd developed more self-esteem growing up, she wouldn't need to depend so much on other people's responsiveness, is a common one. Needing someone to respond to us tempts us to believe that if we were stronger we wouldn't need other people so much. That way they wouldn't be able to disappoint us so much.

Being listened to does help us grow up feeling secure; but, contrary to what some people would like to believe, we never become whole and complete, finished products, like a statue or a monument. On the contrary, like any living thing, human beings require nourishment not only to grow up strong but also to maintain their strength and vitality. Listening nourishes our sense of worth.

The more insecure we are, the more reassurance we need. But all of us, no matter how secure and well adjusted, need attention to sustain us. In case this isn't immediately evident, all you need to do is note how we all have our own preferred ways of announcing our news. If my wife has news, for example, she's likely to call me at work or tell me as soon as she gets home. If she has something to say, she says it. Not me. If I have good news, I hoard it, save it up to announce with a fanfare—dying to be made a fuss over.

I once worked for months trying to land a book contract. My wife knew I was working on the book, but I didn't let her know that a contract was imminent. Waiting and hoping, and trying not to let myself hope for too much, I had extravagant fantasies about getting good news—no, about sharing it. Telling my wife would be the payoff. What I didn't want to do was simply tell her; I wanted—I needed—my announcement to be a big deal. The day the contract finally arrived I was ecstatic. But the best part was looking forward to telling my wife. So I called her at work and told her I had a surprise for her: I was taking her out for a fancy dinner. She said fine and didn't ask any questions. (She's only known me for thirty years.)

By the time I got home, my wife had changed into a silk dress and was ready to go out. She could tell I was excited, but she waited patiently to find out why. At the restaurant, I ordered a bottle of champagne, and when it came she asked, still patient, "Do you have something to tell me?" I pulled out my contract and presented it with all the savoir faire of a ten-year-old showing off his report card. She saw what it was and her face lit up with a huge grin. That look—her love and pride—was indescribably sweet. My own smile was wet with tears.

What elaborate lengths we go to for such moments! Those of us who feel the need to arrange special occasions for our announcements share a good deal with those who don't need to calculate so. The period of time during which we're waiting to tell our news is charged with anxious anticipation. We can feel the tension building. The tension has to do with an aroused impulse—to confess or confront or show off or propose—to make an impact on another person and be responded to. The excitement comes from hope for a positive response; the anxiety comes from fear of rejection or indifference.

Whom you choose to tell what says something about your relationship to yourself—and to the other people in your life. Your presentation of self involves pride and shame—and whom you choose to share them with. With whom do you feel safe to cry? To complain? To rage? To brag? To confess something truly shameful?

• • •

A good listener is a witness, not a judge of your experience.

• • •

As soon as you're able to say what's on your mind—and be heard and acknowledged—you are unburdened. It's like having an ache suddenly relieved. If this completion comes quickly, as it often does in day-to-day conversations, you may hardly be aware of your need for understanding. But the disappointment you feel when you're not heard and the tension you feel waiting and hoping to be heard are signs of how important being listened to is. There are times when all that can be thought must be spoken and heard, communicated and shared, when ignorance and silence are pain, and to speak is to try to alleviate that pain.

"Guess What!"

Remember the last time something really wonderful happened to you. Do you remember waiting to tell someone? Whom did you choose and how did it work out?

Being Heard Means Being Taken Seriously

The need to be heard, which is something we ordinarily take for granted, turns out to be one of the most powerful motives in human nature. Being listened to is the medium through which we discover ourselves as understandable and acceptable—or not. We care about the people who listen to us. We may even love them. But, for a time at least, we use them.

When we're activated by the need for appreciation, we relate to others as *selfobjects*, psychoanalyst Heinz Kohut's telling expression for a responsive other, someone we relate to not as an independent person with his or her own agenda but as someone-there-for-us.[1]

---

[1]Heinz Kohut, *The Analysis of the Self* (New York: International Universities Press, 1971).

Perhaps the idea of using listeners as selfobjects reminds you of those bores who are always talking about themselves and don't seem to care about what you have to say. When they listen, their hearts aren't in it. They're only waiting to change the subject back to themselves.

This lack of appreciation can be especially painful when it occurs between us and our parents. It's maddening when they can't seem to let us be people in our own right, individuals with legitimate ideas and aspirations. Watching our parents listen to other people right in front of us can be especially aggravating. Why don't they show *us* a little of that attention? Here's the writer Harold Brodkey in *The Runaway Soul* dramatizing this irritating experience through the conversation of a young woman and her boyfriend. The boyfriend speaks first:

"Does your dad ever listen, or does he just do monologues?"

"He just does monologues. Doesn't he let you talk?"

"Only if I insist on it. Then we do alternate monologues."

"Well, that's it, then. He talks to you more than he does to me now."

Of course the woman's father talks to her boyfriend more than he does to her. The boyfriend is a fresh audience, new blood.

The people who hurt us most are invariably the ones with whom we think we have a special relationship, who make us feel that our attention and understanding are particularly important to them—until we see how easily they shift their interest to someone else. Right in the middle of confiding in us, they'll catch someone else's eye and break off to talk to that person. We discover that what we thought was an understanding shared only with us is something they've told a dozen people. So much for our special status as confidants! What's so hurtful about these promiscuous "intimates" isn't that they use us, but that they rob us of the feeling that we're important to them, that we're special.

Although none of us likes to see (especially in ourselves) the kind of blatant narcissism that disregards the feelings of others, the truth is, much of the time we're all hopelessly absorbed with ourselves. The subject of narcissism turns out to be crucial in exploring the art of listening. I mention it here only to note that one aspect of our need for other people is entirely selfish. Being listened to maintains our narcissistic equilibrium—or, to put it more simply, it helps us feel good about ourselves.

When Roxanne and her parents finished unloading the car, she felt a sinking sensation and was conscious for the first time of all the things she didn't have. Anxiously she watched as the other students and their families trooped into the dormitory, loaded down with beautiful pillows and down comforters, iPods and DVDs, straightening rods, laptops, tennis rackets, and lacrosse sticks. Roxanne had never even seen a lacrosse stick. By the time her parents drove off, leaving her standing alone in front of South Hall, her excitement about starting college had given way to dread.

Roxanne never did get over her sense of isolation that first year. Everyone else seemed to make friends so easily. Not her. She called home a lot and tried to tell her parents how awful it was. But they said "Don't worry, honey; everybody's a little lonesome at first," and "You should make more friends," and "Maybe you just have to study a little harder." If only it were that easy!

• • •

Reassuring someone isn't the same as listening.

• • •

By the first of December Roxanne was skipping classes, missing meals, and crying herself to sleep. When she couldn't stand it anymore, she made an appointment at the counseling center.

Roxanne was surprised when the therapist said to call her Noreen. She wasn't used to that kind of openness in adults. Noreen turned out to be the most sympathetic person Roxanne had ever met. She didn't tell Roxanne what to do or analyze her feelings; she just listened. For Roxanne, it was a new experience.

With Noreen's help, Roxanne was able to get through that first year and the three years that followed. Noreen helped her discover that her feelings of insecurity stemmed from never feeling really loved by her parents. Roxanne had always thought they were pretty good parents, but she could see now that they never actually knew her very well. Her father was always busy, and her mother never really took her seriously as a person.

Eventually Noreen convinced Roxanne that she would never be free of her anger—and vulnerability to depression—until she worked things out with her parents. When Roxanne agreed, Noreen suggested that she get in touch with me for a few family therapy sessions.

Roxanne and her parents arrived separately for our first meeting, and although they were all smiling, the three of them seemed as wary as cats circling a snake. I had suggested to Roxanne over the phone that we go slow in this first meeting, that she try not to unload the full weight of her anger on her parents but rather search for some common ground. But that wasn't the truth about what she was feeling, and the truth was what she was after. She started in on her father. When she was little, she'd loved him, she said, but as she got older she increasingly saw him as ridiculous and irrelevant. (He worked hard, had a crew cut, voted Republican, and was a patriot. Almost nothing in his life caused him second thoughts.) After listening to his daughter's ungenerous assessment, Roxanne's father said, "So that's how you see me?" and then retreated into silence, his own brand of armor.

Then Roxanne turned to her mother. She called her "shallow," "phony," and—the cruelest thing a child can say to a mother—"interested only in yourself." Roxanne's mother tried to listen but couldn't. "That's not true!" she protested. "Why do you have to exaggerate everything?" This only infuriated Roxanne more, and the two of them lashed back and forth at each other with increasingly shrill voices.

I tried to calm them down but wasn't very successful. Roxanne was hell-bent on communicating—not talking, that old-fashioned process of give-and-take, but communicating—that important development where one insistent family member imparts some critical information to the others, confronting them with "the truth" whether they want to hear it or not. Roxanne's mother left the session in tears.

The following week I met with Roxanne alone. She was sorry the meeting hadn't gone better but was glad to have gotten her feelings out. She thought her mother had shown herself to be the unaccepting person Roxanne knew her to be. They weren't on speaking terms, and that was just fine with Roxanne.

Six months later, much to my surprise, Roxanne called to say that she and her parents wanted to come for another meeting. This time the conversation was friendly but superficial. Roxanne complimented her mother on her shoes and asked about her younger sister. Her mother asked Roxanne how she was doing. Had she gotten over all that bitterness? Roxanne, feeling once again patronized and dismissed, tried to avoid reacting but couldn't. Furiously, she accused her mother of not really being interested in how she was feeling and caring only about polite formalities. My heart sank. But this time Roxanne's mother didn't react angrily or cut her daughter off. She didn't say much, but she didn't interrupt to defend herself either. What enabled her to listen to her daughter's angry accusations this time? I don't know. But she did.

One of a mother's heaviest burdens is being the target of her children's primitive swings between need and rage. The rage is directed at the hand that rocks the cradle no matter how loving its care. It's part of breaking away. Roxanne's mother seemed to sense this, seemed to remember that her daughter was still a little girl in some ways.

Roxanne seemed to expect retaliation from her mother. But when it wasn't forthcoming, she calmed down considerably. She had wanted, it seemed, only to be heard.

After that, Roxanne's relationship with her family changed dramatically. Previously limited to monologues or muteness, they entered into dialogue. Roxanne phoned and wrote. She shared confidences with her mother. Not always, of course, and not always successfully, but Roxanne had become more open to her mother as a person, rather than perceiving her simply as a mother, who was somehow supposed to make everything right. She, in turn, became less a child and more a young woman, ready for life on her own.

Roxanne's unfulfilled need to be listened to had cut her off from other people and filled her with resentment. Unburdening herself was like breaking down a wall that had kept her from feeling connected to other people. That her feelings were somewhat infantile says only that they were a long time unspoken. Talking to Noreen, who didn't have a stake in defending herself, helped Roxanne find her voice.

That second meeting with Roxanne and her parents had produced one of those moments that happen once in a while in families, when someone says something and everything shifts. Only it wasn't what Roxanne said that caused the shift; she'd said it all before. It was that her mother put aside her own claims to being right and just listened.

When we learn to hear the unspoken feelings beneath someone's anger or impatience, we discover the power to release the bitterness that keeps people apart. With a little effort, we can hear the hurt behind expressions of hostility, the resentment behind avoidance, and the vulnerability that makes people afraid to speak or truly listen. When we understand the healing power of listening, we can even begin to listen to things that make us uncomfortable.

Being heard means being taken seriously. It satisfies our need for self-expression and our need to feel connected to others. The receptive listener allows us to express what we think and feel. Being heard and acknowledged helps us clarify both the thoughts and the feelings, in the process firming our sense of ourselves. By affirming that we are understandable, the listener helps confirm our common humanity. Not being listened to makes us feel ignored and unappreciated, cut off and alone. The need to be known, to have our experience understood and accepted by someone who listens, is food and drink to the human heart.

Without a sufficient amount of sympathetic understanding in our lives, we're haunted by an amorphous unease that leaves us anxious and lonely. Such feelings are hard to tolerate, and so we seek solace in passive escapism; we snap on the TV, treat ourselves to Ben and Jerry's, or escape into popular fiction about people whose lives are exciting. There is, of course, nothing wrong with relaxing. But why do we turn on the TV even when there's nothing to watch? And why do we feel restless without the car radio playing, even when it's just noise?

We usually associate passive escapism with release from stress. While it's true that many of us feel used up at the end of the day, it may not be overwork that wears us down, but a lack of understanding in our lives. Chief among the missing elements is the attention and appreciation of responsive selfobjects, people who care and listen to us with interest. When the quality of our relationships isn't sufficient to maintain our equilibrium and enthusiasm—or when we're not up to making them so—we seek escape from morbid self-consciousness. We seek stimulation, excitement, responsiveness, gratification—the same kinds of feelings that can be had from a heart-to-heart talk with someone we care about. But without the ballast of someone to talk to, some of us will continue to drown out the silence, as though without some kind of electronic entertainment to distract us, we may hear the low rumblings of despair.

Exercises

1. Who is the best listener you know? What makes that person a good listener? (Not interrupting? Asking interested questions? Acknowledging what you've said?) What is being with that person like?

What can you learn from that person that would make you a better listener?

2. What do you hesitate to talk to your partner about? Why? What happens to those withheld thoughts and feelings? What are the consequences of that withholding for you? For the relationship?

3. If you improved the way you listen, who would you want to notice? What conversations would you like to go differently?

4. If people think you aren't listening to them, what will they assume it means? What will this lead to?

5. If people think you are listening to them, what will they assume it means? What will this lead to?

6. The next time something is really bothering you, notice how you feel about wanting to talk with someone. Does something hold you back? What do you worry about? If you do share your feelings with someone, what happens?

2

...

"Thanks for Listening"

How Listening Shapes Us
and Connects Us to Each Other

We define and sustain ourselves in conversation with others. Recognition—being listened to—is the response from another person that makes our experience meaningful. It allows us to realize our own agency and authorship in a tangible way. But, as we saw in Chapter 1, the expression and recognition so fundamental to our well-being is a mutual, reciprocal process. Our lives are coauthored in conversation. So, if being recognized through listening is to define and sustain us, it must come from someone whom we in turn recognize. Striking a balance between expression (talking) and recognition (listening) is what allows us and the people we care about to interact as sovereign equals.

If your life, or even a key relationship in it, is unbalanced—if it doesn't allow you sufficient self-expression and mutual recognition—you will be the poorer for it. Listening is critical to the formation of a strong and healthy self *and* to the formation of strong and healthy relationships.

What makes listening such a force in shaping character is the power of words to match and share experience—or contradict and falsify it. What is understood and accepted—"Yes, isn't that wonderful!"—becomes part of the social self, the self you own and share. What doesn't get appreciated—"You shouldn't be feeling that way in the first place"—becomes part of the private self, known but not shared, or disowned, kept secret, sometimes even from yourself. Ominously, much of what fails to find acceptance becomes part of the disavowed self, what psychoanalyst Harry Stack Sullivan called the "not me."[1] Some parents may be too anxious to tolerate a child's anger; others may be too embarrassed to tolerate their children's sexual feelings. Each of us grows up with some experiences of self so poisoned with anxiety that they aren't assimilated into the rest of our personality. Listening shapes us; not being heard twists us.

A young mother in denim was berating her little girl for wanting a Barbie doll. It was a *stupid* thing to want; the child *should be ashamed of herself*; she *should have more self-respect*. It was painful to hear. The sad irony of a mother hammering away at a little girl's pride to teach her self-respect was hard to escape. Should a mother let her daughter have a Barbie, like all the other kids? That's up to her; but she should respect her daughter's right to have opinions of her own.

Gradually, with cooperation between parent and child, a self is formed, organized by language and listening, based in part on the child's natural experience, in part on the values imposed by the parents. The listened-to child grows up whole and secure. The unlistened-to child lacks the understanding that firms self-acceptance and is "bent out of shape" by the wishes and anxieties of others. This is what psychotherapist Carl Rogers meant when he said that the child's innate tendency toward self-actualization is subverted by the need to please.[2]

• • •

**What never gets heard affects more than the difference
between the socially shareable and the private; it drives
a split between the true self and a false self.**

• • •

The seeds of listening are sown in childhood, in the quality of the relationship between parent and child. Parents who listen make their children feel worthwhile and appreciated. Being listened to helps build

[1]Harry Stack Sullivan, *The Interpersonal Theory of Psychiatry* (New York: Norton, 1953).
[2]Carl Rogers, *Client-Centered Therapy* (Boston: Houghton-Mifflin, 1951).

a secure self, endowing a child with sufficient self-respect to develop his or her own unique talents and ideals and to approach relationships with confidence.

That understanding builds self-assurance is hardly news. Most of us can picture a mother with smiling eyes listening enthusiastically to a child eagerly describing some triumph or a father comforting a sad-faced child crying over some minor tragedy. And we all know how bad it feels to watch a parent reduce a child to tears of humiliation for making a mistake. Of course such scenes, repeated over and over, have an impact on a child. What may not be so obvious is how early or how profoundly the quality of listening begins to shape character.

How Listening Shapes Self-Respect

To begin with, the self is not a given, like having red hair or being tall, but a perspective on awareness, and an interpersonal one at that. The self is how we personify what we are, as shaped by our experience of being responded to by others. Character is formed in relationships, and the vitality of the self depends on the quality of listening we receive.

Among scientific findings with the most profound implications for understanding the importance of listening is the work of infant researcher Daniel Stern.[3] Stern's most radical discovery was that the infant is never totally undifferentiated (symbiotic) from the mother.

Margaret Mahler's influential theory of separation and individuation was based on the assumption that we grow up and out of relationships, rather than becoming more active and sovereign *within* them.[4] But once we accept the idea that we don't begin life as part of an undifferentiated unity, the question isn't how we separate from our parents but how we learn to connect. The challenge isn't to become free of people, but to make ourselves understood in relationship to them.

This view of the self as having a fundamental need for expression and recognition emerged not only from the observation of infants but also in consulting rooms, where psychotherapists hear the child's cry in the adult

---

[3]Daniel Stern, *The Interpersonal World of the Infant* (New York: Basic Books, 1985).

[4]Margaret Mahler, Fred Pine, and Anni Bergman, *The Psychological Birth of the Human Infant* (New York: Basic Books, 1975).

voice. The anguish of those who feel empty and alone, unable to connect to other people, leads to the question "What does it take to make us feel whole?" A large part of the answer is being listened to.

In charting the development of children, Stern identified four progressively more complex senses of self, each defining a different domain of self-experience and social relatedness. Second only to the need for food and shelter is the need for understanding. Even infants need listening to thrive. "Listening" to an infant may sound somewhat stilted, but it is precisely that—the quality of parental responsiveness—that plays such a decisive role in making us what we are.

Let's look now at the unfolding of these four senses of self to see how listening shapes character.

"Here I Am.": The Sense of an Emergent Self (Birth to Two Months)

The infant's need for listening is simple but imperative. With the sudden pressure of physical need, life goes from lovely to all wrong. Hunger breaks over the body like an angry storm. It starts slowly; the baby has a sense of something going awry. Then fussing turns to full-throated crying as the baby tries to hurl the pain sensations out and away. This crying serves as a distress signal, like a siren, to alert the parents and demand a response from them.

Being a parent at this stage is simple. As I recall, my wife and I, our empathic sensitivities honed to razor sharpness by months of sleep deprivation, were flung into action by the slightest peep. Blessed with a disposition as placid as a howler monkey, our first little darling would ever so gently summon us for her nightly lactose intolerance test. I, never the insensitive father, was usually first to respond. "Honey," I'd coo, grinding my teeth to keep them warm, "do something!" At which my mate, ever appreciative of my support, would hasten to the little one's side to administer whatever first aid was required. Ah, parenthood.

Babies are cute and helpless, but their smiling, fretting, and crying are commanding messages; they must be listened to. At this stage parents, thinking primarily about satisfying the baby's needs, may not recognize the extent of the social interaction involved in the process. But even before the baby achieves self-consciousness, parents invest it with their expectations and aspirations. From day one, they relate to the baby as both an actual and a potential self.

Our impulse toward understanding is irresistible. Developmental psychologist Aidan Macfarlane's observations of new mothers talking to their infants for the first time after delivery show that the mothers attribute meaning to each sign and sound.[5] "What's that frown for? The world's a little scary, huh?" Mothers don't really believe the infant understands, but they assign meaning to what their infants are doing and respond accordingly. In time, they create little formats of interaction, jointly constructed little worlds. This is the child's first culture.

Parents immediately ascribe intentions to their babies ("Oh, you want that"), motives ("You're doing that so Mommy will hurry up and feed you"), and authorship of action ("You did that on purpose, didn't you?"). In so doing, parents are responding to and helping create an emergent self. Such motives and intentions make human behavior understandable, and parents invariably treat their infants as understandable beings—that is, as the people they are to become (just so long as they become the people their parents want them to become).

• • •

Who we are and what we say triggers other people's response to us. That response and our connection to others remain vital to our psychological well-being.

• • •

When babies are too young to talk, their parents have to understand what they feel but cannot say. When a baby cries, the parents must figure out what's wrong. Does he want to be fed? Does she need a diaper change? Does he want to be held? (Imagine the baby's feelings. What a chasm separates her from these two giant, nervous creatures nature has assigned as her waitpersons. Would they ever catch on?) When the baby grows up and learns to talk, she becomes better at putting her needs and feelings into words. Better, but not perfect. Sometimes we all need a little help making ourselves understood.

---

[5] Aiden Macfarlane, *The Psychology of Childbirth* (Cambridge, MA: Harvard University Press, 1977).

Infants are helplessly dependent on their parents. When the parents are absent, angry, or otherwise unresponsive, the child is alone and terrified; he feels the bottom dropping out of his whole world. This primal connection to others begins as a matter of life and death, over which we have little control when we're infants. Gradually we become aware of our own half of the equation (some people more gradually than others).

Okay, so it's been a while since you depended on your parents to hear your cries and recognize that you were a person with needs and feelings. What significance does this stage of dependence on being heard have for us as adults?

Unlike infants, we don't have to be listened to in order to know that we are persons—existential agents who are initiators of actions. But what listening does provide for us as adults is an opportunity to articulate and integrate deeper layers of ourselves. Attention and appreciation on the part of a listener create an interpersonal experience in which we open up and experience a fuller version of ourselves. The experience of being listened to promotes an unfolding of aspects of experience that may have been closed off because they were never vitalized by being shared and acknowledged. For an infant, being listened to helps confirm that he or she is a self. For an adult, being listened to helps that developmental process to continue—enabling us to provide a fuller account of ourselves and a fuller acceptance of our multidimensional selves.

Adrienne had been going with Phillip for three years when she met Cliff. She hadn't made any promises to Phillip, but they'd been together so long that she didn't really feel okay about seeing another guy. After about a month of wondering what to do, she finally talked to her friend Judy.

Judy had been married long enough to know that you never know how relationships are going to turn out. So when Adrienne told her about Cliff, she just listened. She asked a few questions, like what did Adrienne want, what was she afraid of, and what did she hope would happen, but mostly she just allowed Adrienne to talk.

Adrienne didn't make any final decisions as a result of that conversation, but she did get a lot clearer about what she wanted. She knew she didn't want to be alone, but she wasn't ready to get tied down, either. Phillip was a genuinely nice guy, but she wasn't really in love with him. Cliff was more exciting, but she wasn't sure he was the kind of person she could count on. She was happy to have Phillip in her life, but since she didn't think she wanted to spend the rest of her life with him, she wasn't willing to close off other options. If she saw Cliff occasionally without breaking up with Phillip, there might be complications, but she was willing to risk them.

Sometimes in injury or illness we revisit our childhood feelings of dependency. At times like these our need for other people is self-evident and we experience their response to us as validating our experience or not.

When Valerie got one of those migraines that struck without warning, she told her husband that she couldn't go out to dinner because she had a headache. He said he was sorry she didn't feel well and suggested that she take some aspirin and lie down. Aspirin didn't work for her, and she'd rather stay downstairs and put an ice pack on her forehead. Shouldn't he know that by now? Valerie was glad not to have to go out, but she felt that her husband's suggestion to go upstairs and lie down was just pushing her away. He liked going out to dinner with her, liked having her go to the gym with him, liked having her listen to his problems and accomplishments, but it didn't seem like he was willing to be with her when she didn't feel well.

Most of us eventually grow up, but we never outgrow the need to be taken seriously—to have our feelings recognized.

"Hey, Look at Me!": The Sense of a Core Self (Two to Seven Months)

Between eight and twelve weeks, infants become gregarious. The social smile emerges; they begin to vocalize and make eye-to-eye contact. When the baby looks up and smiles and coos, or splashes in the bath, or giggles with delight, how could you *not* love her? Surely, we would like to think, all parents respond intuitively to such communications. Unfortunately, that isn't so. Some parents are so preoccupied, depressed, or otherwise distracted that they ignore their babies. And, perhaps more common, many parents respond to their babies not as little people with their own rhythms and moods but as foils for the parents' needs.

Every infant has an optimal level of excitement. Activity beyond that level constitutes overstimulation, and the experience becomes upsetting; below that level, stimulation is, well, unstimulating. Parents must learn to read their babies. By taking their children seriously as persons, responding to the children's feelings rather than imposing their own, parents convey acceptance that children take in and transform into self-respect.

The next time you see an adult interacting with a baby, notice the difference between responding in tune with the child's level of excitement and imposing the adult's emotions on the child. When you see a parent with blunted emotions ignoring a bright-eyed baby, you're witnessing the beginning of a long, sad process by which unresponsive parents wither the enthusiasm of their children like unwatered flowers.

Having quite enough unwatered flowers at the office, thank you, I wasn't about to have any around my house. I remember tiptoeing into the baby's room at eventide, right about the time she was dozing—or pretending to. What my masculine intuition told me she really wanted was not rest but to be hurled violently up to the ceiling and then come crashing toward the floor—like a skydiver without a parachute—only to be plucked from the jaws of death by Daddy. Whee!

Too choked with joy to speak, the little mite showed her pleasure by widening her eyes like saucers while her face turned a lovely shade of blue.

Excessive enthusiasm may be less depressing, but it isn't necessarily more responsive. We've all seen grown-ups at it—"baby love"—the fulsome tone of voice, the honeyed words, the endless marveling and exclaiming. When babies are little, it's almost automatic; babies are so animated themselves that they drive up the intensity of our response. But when this adult enthusiasm exceeds the baby's own, the result is a jarring discontinuity. Loving parents share the moods of their children and show it.

• • •

It isn't exuberance or any other emotion that conveys loving appreciation, it's being understood, and taken seriously.

• • •

The baby whose parents tickle and poke and jiggle and shake her when she's not in the mood is as alone with her real self as the baby whose parents ignore her. This imposition of the parents' agenda is, in what psychiatrist R. D. Laing so tellingly called the "politics of experience," the mystification in which the child's reality gets lost.[6] Not being understood and taken seriously as a person in your own right—even at this early age—is the root of aloneness and insecurity. In the words of psychoanalyst Ernest Wolf, "Solitude, psychological solitude, is the mother of anxiety."[7]

Eleanor appreciates getting flowers from her children on Mother's Day but wishes they'd find time to call more often.

Ted tells Katie that he's worn out and wants to stay home and watch a movie on TV. Katie says that maybe he'd feel better if they went out for a walk.

Nikki tells her father about an older colleague at work who often interrupts her at staff meetings. She doesn't want to make a fuss, but she wants to be able to finish saying what's on her mind. Her father tells her that the next time he does that, she should tell him to shut up, she's not finished. Nikki thanks him and changes the subject.

What these examples have in common is that when people respond to us in terms of their own preferences rather than tuning in to ours, it feels like they don't really know us, don't really get who we are—aren't really listening.

"Honey, I'm Cold. Don't You Want a Sweater?": The Sense of a Subjective Self (Seven to Fifteen Months)

By about one year of age the baby realizes that she has an inner, private mental world, with desires, feelings, thoughts, and memories, which are invisible to others unless she makes an attempt to reveal them. The pos-

---

[6] R. D. Laing, *The Politics of Experience* (New York: Pantheon, 1967).

[7] Ernest Wolf, "Developmental Line of Self-Object Relations," in Arnold Goldberg, ed., *Advances in Self Psychology* (New York: International Universities Press, 1980).

sibility of sharing these invisible contents of the mind is the source of the greatest human happiness and frustration.

Imagine for a moment that you're a baby who hasn't yet learned to talk, and you want a cookie. What do you do if you see the cookie but it's out of reach? Simple. You get your mother to read your mind.

Mind reading may sound extravagant, but isn't that what communication boils down to? The baby must gain Mother's attention, express what's on his mind, and do so in a way that Mother receives and understands the message.

"I want a cookie" is a simple message, easily sent and easily received, even without words. When it comes to more complicated messages, babies (like you and me) may have to work harder to express themselves—and hope their listeners will work hard enough to understand.

The possibility of sharing experience creates the possibility for confirmation of the self as understandable and acceptable; it also creates the possibility of intimacy, fulfilling the desire to know and be known. What's at stake is nothing less than discovering what part of the private world of inner experience is shareable and what part falls outside the pale of commonly accepted human experience.

• • •

Being listened to spells the difference between feeling accepted and feeling isolated.

• • •

The possibility of sharing mental states between people also raises the possibility of misunderstanding. For example, babies are remarkably eager explorers. Sitting on Mommy's or Daddy's lap, a baby may probe the parent's mouth or nose with a finger or tug at a strand of hair to see if it will come loose. The parent who takes this exploration as an act of aggression may get annoyed and attribute hostility to the baby. If so, the parent may follow up this feeling with a rebuke, a slap, or some rejection of the baby, who had only been doing what comes naturally at this age.

The misunderstood baby is confused by the parent's lack of understanding, upset and frightened by the rebuke. *Maybe it was a mistake*, the baby thinks. Then, if the baby repeats the exploration, to clarify the confusion or to evoke a different response this time, the baby may now do so with a more energetic assertiveness. Now the parent will assume that his or her original misunderstanding was confirmed: the baby *is* being aggressive.

If this situation is repeated, the parent's false interpretation may become the infant's (and later the child's) official and accepted one: exploration is aggression, and it's bad. The baby may come to see himself as aggressive, even hostile. Someone else's reality has become his. Misunderstanding undermines not only our trust in others, but also our trust in our own perceptions.

The word for sharing experience is *intersubjectivity*. The reason for this fancy term where an ordinary word like *communication* might do is to keep us from forgetting that understanding is a joint achievement: one person trying to express what's on his or her mind, the other trying to read it. Reading a child's mind begins with *attunement*.

Attunement, a parent's ability to share the child's affective state, is a pervasive feature of parent–child interactions with profound consequences. It's the forerunner of empathy and the essence of human understanding. Attunement begins with the intuitive parental response of sharing the baby's mood and showing it. The baby reaches out excitedly and grabs a toy. When the toy is in her grasp, she lets out an exuberant "aah!" and looks at her mother. Mother responds in kind, sharing the baby's exhilaration and showing it by smiling and nodding and saying "Yes!" The mother has understood and shared the child's mood. That's attunement.

One demonstration of the baby's need for an attuned response is the *still-face procedure*. If a mother (or father) goes still-faced—impassive and expressionless—in the middle of an interaction, the baby will become upset and withdraw. Infants after about two-and-a-half months of age react strongly to this still face. They look about. Their smile dies away and they frown. They make repeated attempts to reignite the mother by smiling and gesturing and calling her. If they don't succeed, they finally turn away, looking unhappy and confused.[8] It hurts to reach out to someone who doesn't respond.

"No, I Don't Want a Nap! I Want to Play.": The Sense of a Verbal Self (Fifteen to Eighteen Months)

Learning to speak creates a new type of connection between parent and child. The acquisition of language has traditionally been seen as a major step in the achievement of a separate identity, next only to locomotion.

---

[8]Daniel Stern, *Diary of a Baby* (New York: Basic Books, 1990).

But the opposite is also true: the acquisition of language is a potent force for interaction and intimacy.

Developmental psychologists Arnold Sameroff and Robert Emde summarize an extensive literature that shows that emotional unresponsiveness produces an infant with "a restricted range of emotional expressiveness; less clear signaling; and a predominance of disengagement, distress, or avoidance in interactions. Under these conditions, clinicians may also see a 'turning off' of affective interactions and, in extreme cases, sustained sadness or depression."[9] In other words, a child whose communications aren't appreciated and responded to eventually gives up and turns inward.

● ● ●

When we see sadness or depression in someone, we tend to assume that something's wrong, that something's happened. Maybe that something is that nobody's listening.

● ● ●

The Listened-To Child Is a Confident Child

By the time children get to be four or five, empathy or its absence has molded their personalities in recognizable ways. The securely understood child grows up to expect others to be available and receptive. This is demonstrated by a tendency to draw effectively on preschool teachers as resources. The listened-to child who becomes ill or injured at school will confidently turn to teachers for support. In contrast, it's particularly at such times that insecure children fail to seek contact. "A boy is disappointed and folds his arms and sulks. A girl bumps her head under a table and crawls off to be by herself. A child is upset on the last day of school; she sits frozen and expressionless on a couch."[10] Such reactions are typical—and don't change much as the unlistened-to child gets older.

Preschoolers with a history of empathic listening are more engaged and more at ease with their peers. They expect interactions to be positive and thus are more eager for them. They are able to make more friends and

[9] Arnold Sameroff and Robert Emde, eds., *Relationship Disturbances in Early Childhood* (New York: Basic Books, 1989), p. 47.

[10] Alan Sroufe, "Relationships, Self, and Individual Adaptation," in Arnold Sameroff and Robert Emde, eds., *Relationship Disturbances in Early Childhood* (New York: Basic Books, 1989), pp. 88–89.

are happier. They are also good listeners. Already by four or five, empathic failure—not abuse or cruelty, but simple, everyday lack of understanding—results in a self that is isolated and insecure, vulnerable to rejection and therefore fearful of new people and experience.

"He Never Talks to Me."

The reticence of some men may have as much to do with a history of not being empathically responded to as to anything inherent about gender. Getting uncommunicative people to open up requires an extra effort to demonstrate acceptance of their feelings—including feeling like not talking about something right now.

Imagine five-year-old Tammy, weaned on understanding, telling her playmate about a bully in kindergarten. "And then he pushed me and hogged all the crayons!"

A tiny cloud momentarily overshadowed her friend Ryan's even tinier face. Bullies were not his favorite people. But listening sympathetically, he knew, was for sissies. Confident that if his own ire were sufficiently aroused, he could demolish a grape with a single blow of his fist, Ryan counseled war. "You should put paint in his hair and spank him with your ruler when he does that."

Here were two kindred spirits, meeting at last on a plane of perfect understanding. "Thanks," said Tammy gratefully, "but I think I hear my mother calling. Nice talking to you."

The need for listening is based partly on the need to sustain our sense of significance. The listener's understanding presence serves a selfobject function—to satisfy our need for attention and appreciation. But the idea that listening is something one person *gives* to the other is only partly true. Another vital aspect of listening is mutuality.

Listening Bridges the Space Between Us

Mutuality is a sense not merely of being understood but of sharing—of being-with another person. Here it isn't just *I* but *we* that is important. Our experience is made fuller by sharing it with another person.

When I want to "share" a thought or feeling that means a lot to me, what I want is to be understood, taken seriously and appreciated. (Calling this "sharing" is an unctuous affectation; what we really want is to express ourselves and be heard.) It is I who wants to be validated. But if I see an especially funny cartoon in *The New Yorker*, I immediately think of someone to share it with. (Here, "sharing" is appropriate, because the experience sought is mutual, communal.) In this instance I don't want to be admired or valued; I just want to share the laughter.

As psychologist Ruthellen Josselson says in *The Space Between Us*,[11] mutuality is a powerful but neglected aspect of human experience. When we're young and alive, before life blunts our naked nerve endings, the yearning for mutuality takes its most intense form in the hungering for a soul mate. We find or invent a special someone with whom we can share light moments and deep thoughts.

Mutuality is the stuff of everyday human exchange. We swap knowing comments about the president's latest gaffe, complain about the weather, and chat idly about the events of the day. Nothing important is happening, just life and shared humanity. One woman said, "That's why when I'm away on business I call my husband at the end of the day—to tell him that the meeting went okay or it's raining or I forgot to pack my good shoes." This woman doesn't *need* anything; she calls just to share the everyday observations and opinions and complaints that otherwise back up and burden us in isolation.

Most theories of human relationship emphasize one or another aspect of connection, whether it's mutuality, the selfobject function, holding, attachment, or caring. All these many modes of relatedness are ways of reaching through the space that separates us. Underlying all our agendas, however, is the fact that speech is the primary mode of relating, and being listened to is the primary means of being understood and appreciated. By "appreciated" I don't mean admired, but rather perceived and accepted as we feel ourselves to be. When we talk about being down in the dumps, it doesn't help to be told how wonderful we are; we want our discontent recognized. We want to be known.

As we're reminded from time to time when we're misjudged or hurt more than anyone realizes, no one can really see our selves. They see what

---

[11]Ruthellen Josselson, *The Space Between Us: Exploring the Dimensions of Human Relationships* (San Francisco: Jossey-Bass, 1992).

they can and are willing to see, and they know what we tell them. The rest is private, mystery.

The way we become known is through empathic responsiveness, what Heinz Kohut called "mirroring."[12] The good listener (or "mirroring selfobject") appreciates us as we are, accepting the feelings and ideas that we express as they are. In the process, we feel understood, acknowledged, and accepted.

Empathy—the human echo—is the indispensable stuff of emotional well-being. What is adequately mirrored becomes, in time, part of the true and lived self. The child who is heard and appreciated has a better chance to grow up whole. The adult who is heard and appreciated is more likely to continue to feel that way.

Unshared Thoughts Diminish Us

Some people are good at getting appreciated, but they work too hard at it. They aren't open to all of themselves, and so what gets appreciated is only the face they show to the world. Reassurance isn't very reassuring to the person with too many secrets.

Why, then, do some people say so little about themselves?

The answer is, life teaches them to hold back. The innocent eagerness for appreciation we bring to our earliest relationships exposes us to consequences. Some people are lucky. They get the attention they need and thereafter approach life with confidence. Others aren't so lucky. They don't get listened to, and as a consequence they avoid opening up. What might appear to be modesty in some such cases may have more to do with the reluctance to expose old wounds. Many people learn instead to channel their need for appreciation into personal ambition or doing things for other people.

• • •

Not being listened to is hard on the heart, and so to varying degrees we cover our need for understanding with mechanisms of defense.

• • •

---

[12]Kohut's two great (though unfortunately dense) works are *The Analysis of the Self* (New York: International Universities Press, 1971) and *The Restoration of the Self* (New York: International Universities Press, 1977).

Some people become experts at avoidance and cultivate the capacity to be alone. The charm of solitude, celebrated by British psychiatrist Anthony Storr,[13] is that it provides space for repose and reflection, time for looking within the self, time for creative endeavor. Solitude offers respite from the noisy claims of everyday social living. I'll discuss later how solitude can give us a chance to listen to our own thoughts. But some of the penchant for being alone is defensive—an accommodation to being hurt by not being heard. The defenses that form the solitary person's character support a grand illusion: the illusion of self-reliance. If we could only examine the contemplation of one's own feelings that passes for introspection, we'd discover that the silence of the solitary is often filled with imagined conversations.[14]

One of the reasons Sharon found Don so appealing was that he always seemed cool and self-contained. While other people at the office always seemed to be complaining or arguing, Don went about his business with quiet assurance. He never seemed to get into arguments with anyone.

But one morning Sharon couldn't help overhearing a junior colleague come into Don's office and ask if Don was annoyed at her for something. In a barely controlled voice Don said that he didn't care for Ellen's arguing with everything he said in staff meetings. "Oh," she said, sarcastically, "what do you want me to do, agree with everything you say?" At that, Don lost it. He said that she hadn't shown him any respect since she came into the firm; he was sick and tired of her disagreeing with everything he said. She never really considered his ideas, he said in an increasingly shrill voice, she was just being disagreeable. At that point Ellen walked out.

Well, Sharon thought, *I guess Don isn't so self-composed after all. He's just one of those people who stay calm only by avoiding confrontations.*

Unshared thoughts diminish us, not only by making us less authentic and less whole, as we've discussed, but also by eating at us. Repression is not like putting something away on the closet shelf and forgetting about it; repression takes a constant expenditure of energy that slowly wears us down.

---

[13] Anthony Storr, *Solitude: A Return to the Self* (New York: The Free Press, 1988).

[14] In this electronic age, some solitary people retreat to online chat rooms to practice speaking to a safe audience.

The feeling of not being understood is one of the most painful in human experience. Not being appreciated and responded to depletes our vitality and makes us feel less alive. When we're with someone who doesn't listen, we shut down. When we're with someone who's interested and responsive—a good listener—we perk up and come alive. Being listened to is as vital to our enthusiasm for life as love and work. So is being a good listener. Understanding the dynamics of listening enables us to deepen and enrich our relationships. It involves learning how to suspend our own emotional agenda and then realizing the rewards of genuine empathy. When our own listening becomes blocked by the emotions that others arouse in us, we conspire to produce our own isolation. It doesn't have to be that way.

Exercises

1. Is there someone who would love to have you listen more attentively? What gets in the way? If you were to listen more closely to that person, how would it affect your relationship? How would your listening affect how the person feels about you? How would your ability to empathize affect that person's feeling of well-being?

2. Make a list of things that might be worth *not* listening to. These might include always turning the radio on in the car, spending time with people you don't like, snapping on the TV instead of looking out the window, grabbing something to read every time you have a spare few minutes, compulsively listening to music rather than to your own thoughts.

3. Think of someone you avoid telling certain things because of the way that person typically responds to you. Plan in advance to make a gentle comment about that tendency the next time he or she does it.

   N.B. Be prepared to respond without emotionalism if the other person takes umbrage at your comment. The purpose of this exercise is to get you to practice calling people on their annoying listening habits without turning it into a big confrontation. In commenting on their response to you, focus not on what they are doing wrong but on how you prefer to be responded to.

3

• • •

"Why Don't People Listen?"

How Communication Breaks Down

Ellen was finding it more difficult than she'd imagined to stay home all day with two small children. She had planned to go back to work after the children were born but decided that it was more important to be at home with them until they started school. What she missed most about working was having people to talk with. Listening to who wanted a cookie and who had to go to the potty got pretty tedious by the end of the day. Ellen's husband was surprisingly unsympathetic. He helped put the kids to bed and spent time with them on weekends, but when he came home after work he didn't even pretend to be interested in Ellen's account of her day. She was hurt, and she was angry.

"I know Greg works hard and wants to rest. But I work hard too. All I want is a few minutes of adult conversation. But if I dare to interrupt his precious six o'clock news to try to talk to him, he just gets mad. It isn't worth it, and I've had just about all I can take." Her eyes were full of tears.

"Did You Hear What I Said?"

Why don't people listen? There's no shortage of easy answers to that question. Most focus on the listener. (Husbands are notoriously unsympathetic listeners.) Ellen's explanation for Greg's unavailability wasn't completely critical—"I know he needs time to unwind"—but it was, after all, focused entirely on him. His lack of listening was *his* doing.

In fact, listening (or the lack of it) is a two-person process. According to Greg, it was frustrating to talk with Ellen about the kids. "She's always complaining. She says they won't leave her alone, even when she goes to the bathroom. But she encourages it! She won't let them alone to play by themselves, and she refuses to take any time for herself. And the thing that really bothers me is the way she always sides with the younger one. Everything Terri does is cute; everything Cody does is wrong. If I try to say anything, even very nicely, she starts crying and says I'm picking on her. So I've learned to keep my mouth shut."

Ellen felt neglected because Greg wouldn't talk to her, but her contribution to the problem was not being open to his point of view. The fact that Greg's position differs from hers, and may even be critical, makes it hard to hear. Unfortunately, when two people are in conflict about something important, unless each is able to at least acknowledge the other's point of view, the result is likely to be an emotional cutoff.

Greg felt discounted because Ellen complained about a problem of her own making (as he saw it) and wouldn't listen to his opinion. And yet Greg manages neither to listen nor to get his point of view across. If he could separate listening from advising, perhaps Ellen would get some sympathy for her feelings, and then he might be able to communicate his perspective more effectively. Of course it's difficult for him to set aside his own feelings long enough to listen to his wife's, especially on a subject that he feels so strongly about. But maybe that's not a good enough excuse for a husband and father's retreat.

When people don't listen to us, we can't help feeling it's their fault: they're selfish or inconsiderate. (When *we* don't listen, it's because we're bored or tired or don't like being talked down to.) The truth is, listening is a complex process. Even though failures of listening all end in the same painful experience of not being heard, there are many reasons people don't listen.

Several years ago a young couple came to me complaining of difficulties in communicating. When I asked what the problem was, the husband said, "It's my wife; she's boring." (Who says men are reticent with their feelings?) Restraining my urge to react to this nasty crack, I asked him to explain. The man was a lawyer, working as a campaign advisor in a gubernatorial election campaign. His days were filled with strategy sessions, speechwriting conferences, meetings with the candidate, television interviews, arranging appearances across the state, defending attacks from the opposition, and planning counterattacks. When he came home at night, his head spinning from the excitement and frustration of the crusade, he mumbled a greeting to his wife and collapsed onto the couch with a drink and the newspaper.

When I asked why he wasn't more eager to talk over the events of the day, he said his wife wasn't interested. She was a graphic design artist and not at all, he contended, concerned about politics.

She protested that although she might not know a lot about politics, she *was* interested in him and what he was doing. He wasn't convinced.

I asked him to think of someone who he *knew* was interested in the campaign, someone with whom he could talk enthusiastically. Imagine, I told him, how different you are with that person. He allowed as that might be true. Then I asked him—just for an experiment—to come home for one week and pretend that his wife was that interested person, the person he found it so exciting to talk to. He agreed to try it.

The next week they returned beaming. "Guess what?" he said. "She's not boring anymore."

This young lawyer's uncommunicativeness could have been taken as just another example of men's silence. Are men emotionally illiterate? Trapped in doing—working, playing, achieving—do they have no language of feeling? Such stereotyping ignores the interactive nature of communication and the powerful role of expectations. When people don't say much, it's less likely that they have nothing on their minds than that they don't trust the other person to be willing to hear it. My suggestion to this man—that he pretend his wife *was* interested—encouraged him to break his silence. But it was his approaching her with enthusiasm, taking interest in talking to her, that broke the pattern of avoidance. The truth is that we become more interesting when we assume interest on the part of our listeners.

Why Someone Doesn't Hear What You Think You Said

Sometimes people don't hear us because they've had a bad day. They may be preoccupied with the angry things someone said or with all the extra work they have to do. Or they may be turned off to us by any number of things—they assume that we're talking to them only because we want something or that we're going to give them a lecture or that we don't really care about them. Listeners often don't hear because they have a preconceived notion of what we're going to say. Or they can't hear us because they can't suspend their own needs or because what we say makes them anxious. In short, although hurt feelings may tempt us to blame failures of listening on other people's recalcitrance, the reasons for not listening are many and complex.

When the communicative process breaks down, we—who are doing our best—tend to assume that the other person didn't say what he meant or didn't hear what we were saying. Usually, both parties to misunderstanding feel that way. But it may be helpful to realize that between speaker and listener are two filters to meaning.[1]

The speaker, who has an *intention* of what he or she wants to communicate, sends a *message*, and that message has an *impact* on the listener.

Good communication means having the impact you meant to have—that is, *intent* equals *impact*. But every message must pass first through the filter of the speaker's clarity of expression and second through the listener's ability to hear what was said. Unfortunately, there are many times when intent doesn't equal impact and many reasons why this is the case.

Some of the reasons for misunderstanding are simple and can be improved, like learning a skill. For example, by giving feedback, listeners tell speakers about the impact of their messages and give them a chance to clarify their intentions. But many reasons for misunderstanding are less straightforward and not amenable to simple formulas for improvement. Our young lawyer's assumption that his wife wasn't interested in his work is just one example of the psychological complications of listening.

Transference

This dynamic, the speaker's tendency to impose certain expectations on the listener, is what, in the psychoanalytic situation, is called *transference*. For simplicity's sake, the idea of transference is often reduced to the notion that the patient assumes that the silent analyst is a carbon copy of one of

---

[1]John Gottman, Cliff Notarius, Jonni Gonso, and Howard Markman, *A Couples Guide to Communication* (Chicago: Research Press, 1976).

his or her parents, judging her harshly just like her father did or enthralled with his accomplishments the way his mother was. In fact, transference refers to all the ways in which a person's experience of a relationship is shaped by subjectivity—past experience, expectations, sensitivities, hopes, and fears. Transference isn't limited to the therapeutic situation—and it isn't only distortion.

Chris grew up with a jealous and competitive older sister who was always proving him wrong. Chris's sister would ask innocent-sounding questions that always led to the same conclusion: Chris was wrong or dumb, or both. Now whenever Chris's girlfriend asked him a question about something he was explaining, he felt attacked.

• • •

Transference: the way in which a speaker's experience of a listener is unconsciously organized according to preestablished expectations.

• • •

Walter hated his wife's constant criticism. She challenged almost everything he said. Consequently, he didn't say much. According to Julia, Walter was overly sensitive. While he admitted that there might be some truth to that, he insisted that she was a critical and controlling person. "She's always telling me what to do," he said. "She won't leave me alone." If these protests remind you of a teenager complaining about his mother, you're onto something about transference.

Whenever Walter's wife asked him to do something for her, he felt like she was bossing him around. The burden of being cast in the role of a controlling mother is familiar to many women. What to do? This is a tough one. One solution is for the woman to take into account her man's tendency to overreact by carefully avoiding anything that might sound like a complaint. In fact, Walter's wife tried to do just that. Knowing how hypersensitive he was, she'd refrain from asking him anything for weeks at a time. But eventually taking care of the house and yard would get too much for her and she'd complain that she needed him to take some responsibility for the chores. Having waited so long made it hard to keep the annoyance out of her voice. He'd feel scolded and resentful, and the cycle would start all over again.

Another solution is to borrow a technique from Harry Stack Sullivan, founder of the interpersonal school of psychoanalysis. Sullivan was famous for being able to work with severely disturbed patients, many of whom had paranoid delusions (perhaps the most extreme form of projection). Whenever Sullivan feared that a patient might be projecting certain expectations onto him, he'd make what he called "counterprojective comments," explicitly disavowing the role being projected onto him. The point of such comments was to reassure the other person, and so saying, for example, "I'm not your mother!" in a scolding voice would hardly qualify. A more reassuring way to disavow the role of critical mother might be to say "Honey, I don't mean to be critical, but would you do me a favor and not put the cats in the washing machine?"

Transference is usually thought of as distortion. But maybe it also has to do with what the speaker needs from the listener at that moment. Thus, for example, a woman chatting about a program she saw on TV may not impose any particular needs on the person listening to her. On the other hand, if the same woman has just been in an auto accident, she may project onto the listener her need for an empathic selfobject experience. In the first instance, she may enjoy the listener's sharing a similar experience, whereas in the second she may not want to be interrupted except to have her feelings acknowledged.

Countertransference, the psychoanalytic term for the complexity introduced by the listener, refers to how the listener's subjectivity distorts his or her experience of the conversation. Like transference, countertransference isn't simply distortion, because our expectations actually shape and reshape our relationships. The woman who expects men to talk only about themselves may inquire more than she discloses, thereby confirming her expectations. The man who expects to find his wife's account of the day uninteresting may fail to ask the questions that might make it interesting to him; as a result, he gets out of the conversation pretty much what he puts into it.

Dorothy suggested to her brother that they should ask their mother what kind of funeral arrangements she wanted for their father. Ron responded angrily, "Well, I can't just drop everything and fly across the country. I certainly can't stay for a week to sit shivah. I have things to do here and people are counting on me." Dorothy had had no such expectations of her brother and wondered why he had to get so angry at her.

• • •

Countertransference: The listener has an emotional reaction that interferes with hearing what's being said. When listeners are in the grip of countertransference, mature responses, like empathy, perspective, humor, wisdom, and concern for the other person, are distorted through the prism of the listener's emotionality.

• • •

Although the terms transference and countertransference don't really tell you anything you don't already know, they may remind you that listening can be disrupted by either the speaker or the listener. Actually, distinguishing between the two (unless *you* misunderstand something *I've* said) is somewhat arbitrary. The communicative process is always *intersubjective*—that is, it reflects the actions and interactions of both parties' subjective realities.

The principal forces contributing to the listener's filter are the listener's own agenda, preconceived notions and expectations, and defensive emotional reactions.

The Listener's Own Agenda

In the summer of 1992, Ariel Dorfman's play *Death and the Maiden*, starring Glenn Close, Richard Dreyfuss, and Gene Hackman, drew large audiences on Broadway. This play of ideas in the guise of a political thriller takes place in a country that might be Chile in the immediate aftermath of a corrupt dictatorship. The setting is a beach house on the night that the lawyer, Gerardo (Richard Dreyfuss), is asked to investigate political crimes of the recent past, including the rape of his wife, Paulina (Glenn Close). When Roberto Miranda (Gene Hackman) gives her husband a lift home after his tire blows out, she recognizes his voice as that of the doctor who raped her. Paulina gets a gun and ties the doctor to a chair. But her husband doesn't believe her. How could she recognize the man who raped her from just his voice? He can't believe that the good Samaritan who stopped to help him on the road could be the evil man who did such terrible things to his wife. She assures him that she could never forget that voice. Still her husband can't believe her. The play turns on the wife's desperation and the husband's incredulity. The ending is ambiguous.

I first heard about *Death and the Maiden* from a patient who took it as an allegory of a husband's failure to listen to his wife, despite the urgency of her appeal. She knew how the woman felt. I replied that as a metaphor for misunderstanding the story was one-sided, stressing as it did only the husband's failure to listen, rather than also dealing with the wife's failure to make herself understood. I wasn't familiar with the play, but I wanted my patient to quit blaming her husband for their problems and begin to see their communication as a process that took place between them. It wasn't until later that I realized that I was recreating a similar story: a woman was trying to tell a man something—in this case that the play was profoundly disturbing and that it reminded her of not being listened to by her husband—and the man wasn't listening.

When I finally got around to reading the play, I responded the same way my patient did. It's a powerful story about a woman desperate for understanding and desperately not understood.

I didn't listen to my patient with the best of intentions. Oh, I heard what she said all right, but I was too eager to teach her a lesson about listening to really understand what she was saying—that the play was upsetting and reminded her of her own situation. My response, "Yes, but … ," had the effect of making her wrong and me right. Failures of listening often take that form.

To listen well, it's necessary to let go of what's on your mind long enough to hear what's on the other person's. Feigned attentiveness doesn't work.

Remember Roger, whose friend Derek grew distant after he got married? Roger might have been able to talk to Derek if he'd concentrated on saying how he felt, without blaming Derek or forcing him to explain himself. If you can express your feelings without trying to compel anything from the other person, you're more likely to get heard—and more likely to hear what the other person is feeling.

For years, Wayne had trouble listening to Janice's complaining. She was always unhappy about something, and he always felt that she expected him to do something about it. Therefore, because he felt threatened by her complaints, Wayne listened only reluctantly. In fact, when Janice really did want Wayne to do something she would make that perfectly clear. The rest of the time she just had the sense that he wasn't interested in her feelings.

When Janice's mother developed Parkinson's, something shifted in the couple's relationship. Now when Janice talked about the problems she was worried about, Wayne could sympathize because it was clear that he wasn't responsible. He could sense her vulnerability and he felt good about being able to listen and comfort her.

What shifted wasn't the result of anything either of them did deliberately. Wayne became a better listener once he realized he wasn't responsible for doing anything about Janice's feelings, and she became easier to listen to when she expressed her feelings of vulnerability more directly. Too bad it took a crisis to make clear what had always been the case. Wayne wasn't responsible for Janice's feelings, and when she expressed her feelings more directly, he was able to listen. I'll discuss later what you can do to bring about this shift toward mutual understanding, whether you're a listener who gets defensive or a person who has trouble getting people to listen to your feelings.

Preconceived Notions

By the time we emerge from adolescence, most of us have become self-protective. We know where our naked nerve endings are and don't often expose them. We open ourselves selectively and, like any creature with a soft underbelly, retreat from unfriendly encounters. Sometimes, however, it's too late to pull back inside our shells. When the pressure of emotion makes us open ourselves to someone we think we can trust, failed understanding can be as bruising as a mugging.

When his son told him he was dropping out of college, Seth did his best to hide his disappointment. Still, he was upset and needed someone to talk to. Hoping that his brother would understand, Seth gave him a call. It wasn't easy for Seth to talk about his feelings, so he started out making small talk. After a few minutes Seth told his brother that Justin had dropped out of school and that he was very discouraged about it. There was a pause, and then his brother went on to talk about something else. Seth was stunned. How could his brother be so unsympathetic? With great effort, he confronted his brother, saying "Didn't you hear what I said?" His brother replied that he had never thought of Seth as someone who needed emotional support.

Here was a chance for the brothers to share a deeper understanding; if they would only open up and listen to one another, they could reestablish the closeness they'd had so many years ago. But it didn't happen.

The expectations with which we approach others are, as we shall see, just one of many ways we create the listening we get. Nor can the process be reduced to the behavior of the participants—the words—and therefore always be improved by "skills training" or pretending to take an interest or other calculated strategies. (Conversation can, of course, be reduced to a behavioral analysis, but only by trivializing the feelings of the people involved.) Dialogue takes place between two people with not just ears and tongues but hearts and minds—and all the famous complications therein.

• • •

Having an understanding attitude doesn't mean presuming to know a person's thoughts and feelings. It means being open to listening and discovering.

• • •

Emotional Reactivity

As I mentioned in the Introduction, we all have certain ways of reacting emotionally within particular relationships. The closer the relationship, the more vulnerable we are to hearing something said as rejection or attack, even if it wasn't meant that way. Because of the dynamics of the relationship or what we've learned to expect, we get defensive, which makes it impossible to listen to and understand what the speaker meant to say.

A simple "Have you taken the garbage out yet?" might be taken as a rebuke by someone whose parents never expected him to do anything right. His response might be an overreactive "Can't you leave me alone for one second!"

It's not always the listener's defensiveness, of course, that gives rise to heated reactions. Sometimes it's the speaker's provocation.

"Why do I always have to ask you three times before you do anything?" when it really means "Would you please take the garbage out?" will almost inevitably trigger a defensive reaction. For that matter, even "Haven't you taken the garbage out *yet?*" could provoke an emotional response. If you don't watch how you say things as well as what you say, it's easy to provoke those you love.

Then there are those touchy subjects that can almost be counted on to set off an explosion. As I'll explain in Chapters 6 and 9, topics likely to be toxic among couples are money, children, and sex. To have a constructive discussion about any of these, where both people really listen, requires special effort. You might have to watch not only what you say and how you say it but also where, when, and why.

This is not to imply that we need to spend our lives tiptoeing around each other. What it does mean is that we may need to step back and calm down, being aware of what sets us off and what sets off those we want to communicate with, if we are to get through to each other.

When we don't, many exchanges degenerate to such clever repartee as "You're such a bitch!" and "Oh, grow up!" before falling apart altogether as someone storms out of the room.

Understanding the Rules of the Listening Game: Beyond Linear Thinking

We don't usually stop to examine patterns of misunderstanding in our lives because we're stuck in our own point of view. Misunderstanding hurts, and when we're hurt we tend to look outside ourselves for explanations. But the problem isn't just that when something goes wrong we look for someone to blame. The problem is linear thinking. We reduce human interactions to a matter of personalities. "He doesn't listen because he's too self-absorbed." "She's hard to listen to because she goes on and on about everything." Some people blame themselves ("Maybe I'm not that interesting"), but it's usually easier to recognize the other person's contribution.

Attributing other people's lack of understanding to character is armor for ignorance and passivity. That some people repeat their annoying ways with most people they come in contact with doesn't prove that lack of responsiveness is fixed in character; it only proves that these individuals trigger many people to play out the reciprocal role in their dramas of two-part disharmony.

The fixed-character position assumes that it's hard for people to change. But you don't change relationships by changing other people. You change patterns of relating by changing yourself in relation to them. Personality is dynamic, not fixed. The dynamic personality position posits that it is possible for people to change; all we have to do is change our responses to each other. We are not victims—we are participants, in a real way, and the consequences of our participation are profound.

To participate effectively, you have to know something about the rules of the game.

I remember how confused I was the first time I saw a lacrosse game. From where I sat it looked as if some kids were standing around while the rest raced up and down the field, using their sticks to pass the ball back and forth, club each other, or both. I got the gist of it—it was like soccer played by Road Warriors—but a lot of it was hard to follow. Why, for instance, did the team that lost the ball out of bounds sometimes get it back and sometimes not? And why sometimes when one kid whacked another with his stick did everybody cheer, while at other times the referee called a foul? The problem was that I couldn't see the whole field and didn't know the rules of the game.

The same disadvantages—not seeing the whole field and not knowing the rules of the game—keep us from understanding our successes and failures at communicating with one another.

Earlier I said that listening is a two-person process, but even that is oversimplified. Actually, even an uncomplicated communication has several components: the listener, the speaker, the message, various implicit messages, the context, and, because the process doesn't flow one way from speaker to listener, the listener's response. Even a brief consideration of these elements in the listening process reveals more reasons for misunderstanding than simply bad faith on the part of the listener.

"What Are You Trying to Say?"

The message is the point of what a speaker says. But the message sent isn't always the one intended.

A family of four is invited to spend Sunday afternoon at the lake house of friends of the father. When the teenage daughter asks if she can bring along a friend, her father says, "I don't think we should bring extra guests when we're invited to dinner." The daughter looks hurt, and the man's wife says, "You're being silly; they never mind extra company." The man gets angry and withdraws, brooding over his feeling that his wife always takes the children's side and never listens to him.

The problem here is a common one: the message sent wasn't the one intended. One of the unfortunate things we learn along with being "polite" and not being "selfish" is not to say directly what we want. Instead of saying "I want ... ," we say "Maybe we should ... " or "Do you want ... ?" When we're taking a trip in the car and we get hungry, we say "Isn't it getting late?" (When I was growing up I learned that guests weren't supposed to put people to any trouble. If you went to someone's house and wanted a glass of water, you didn't ask; you looked thirsty. If they offered you something, you politely declined. Only if they insisted was it okay to accept. A really good boy waited until a glass of water was offered at least twice before accepting.)

Because this convention of indirectness is so universal, it doesn't usually cause problems. If the other person in the room says "Are you cold?" you can assume he means "Can we turn up the heat?" But indirectness can cause problems when stronger feelings are involved. The father in our example didn't want his daughter to bring a friend. Perhaps his wife was right; the people who invited them wouldn't mind. But somehow *he* minded. Maybe he wanted his daughter to remain more a part of the family and less an independent person with friends of her own. Or maybe he wanted her to be part of the grownups' conversation, instead of off with her friend, because he found it easier to talk about the children's doings than his own. That's the trouble with being indirect: there are always a lot of *maybes*.

When we're conflicted over certain of our own needs, we may infer (rightly or wrongly) that others would object to even hearing our wishes, much less acceding to them. Because indirectness leads to so much misunderstanding, it does more harm than good. Two people can't have an honest disagreement about whether or not they want to move to another city as long as they engage in diversionary arguments about whether going or staying would be better for the children.[2]

One reason others argue with us in a way that seems to negate our feelings is that we blur the distinction between our feelings and the facts. Instead of saying "I don't want her to bring a friend," the father tries to cloud his motives and bolster his argument by appealing to *shoulds*. When his wife argues with what he says instead of what he means, he feels rejected.

● ● ●

Like every listener, he measured the intentions of other speakers by what they said—or what he heard—and asked that they measure him by what he meant to say.

● ● ●

As speakers we want to be heard—not merely listened to—we want to be understood, heard for what we think we're saying, for what we know we meant. Similar impasses occur when we insist we said one thing and our listener heard another. Instead of saying "What I meant to say was ... ," we go on insisting what we *did* say.

"Why Don't You Say What You Mean?"

Implicit messages tell us more than what's being said; they tell us how we're meant to receive what's being said. Depending on the situation, "Let's have lunch" could mean "I'm hungry," "I'd like to see you again," "No, I don't want to go to dinner with you," or "Please leave now; I'm busy." The statements "I love you" and "I'm sorry" are notorious for having multiple meanings. Knowing the other person can make it easier to decode implicit messages; speculating about his or her motives can make it harder.

According to Gregory Bateson, one of the founders of family therapy, all communications have two levels of meaning: *report* and *command*.[3] The

---

[2]There are times, however, when the most effective statement of what you want is less than completely candid. For people who have trouble saying no, rather than trying to explain why they don't want to do something, it may be easier to say "I'd love to, but I can't."

[3]Jurgen Ruesch and Gregory Bateson, *Communication: The Social Matrix of Psychiatry* (New York: Norton, 1951).

report (or message) is the information conveyed by the words. The second or command level (which Bateson called *metacommunication*) conveys information about how the report is to be taken and a statement of the nature of the relationship.

If a wife scolds her husband for running the dishwasher when it's only half full and he says okay but turns around and does the same thing two days later, she may be annoyed that he doesn't listen to her. She means the message. But maybe he didn't like the metamessage. Maybe he doesn't like her telling him what to do as though she were his mother.

In attempting to define the nature of our relationships we qualify our messages by posture, facial expression, and tone of voice. For example, a rising inflection on the last two words turns "You did that on purpose" from an accusation to a question. The whole impact of a statement may change depending on which words are emphasized. Consider the difference between "Are *you* telling me it isn't true?" and "Are you telling me it *isn't* true?" Pauses, gestures, and gaze also tell us how to interpret what's being said. Although we may not need the ponderous term *metacommunication*, misunderstandings about how messages should be taken is a major reason for problems in listening.

One winter when I was working hard and feeling sorry for myself, I wrote to a sympathetic friend and said jokingly that I was running away to spend two weeks on the white beaches of a deserted Caribbean island. The only trouble was that I didn't *say* it, I *wrote* it, and she missed the irony I intended. The medium didn't carry my tone of voice or the facial expression that modified the message. Instead of getting the sympathy I was (indirectly) asking for, I got back a rather testy note saying that it's nice to know that some people have the time and money to indulge themselves.

We know what we mean; problems arise when we expect others to. How is our communication to be taken? Is it chat? A confession? An outpouring of emotion? When our listeners fail to grasp that we're upset and need to have our feelings listened to, who's to blame?

A woman told her husband that something her boss said made her afraid she might be in for trouble at work. The husband responded by saying no, he didn't think so; it didn't sound that way. When she replied that he didn't listen to her, both of them got upset. She was annoyed because he didn't listen to her feelings. He was hurt because he *was* listening. He just didn't realize how upset she was.

Perhaps to some people this woman's upset would have been apparent. Maybe a friend would have realized that she needed to have her feelings acknowledged, not disagreed with. But she wasn't married to that friend. She was married to a man who didn't automatically understand how she wanted to be listened to. (Some people try to make that clear: "I'm worried about something, and I need to talk about it." "I need some advice." "I just need you to listen.")

E-mail makes correspondence so easy that people often send messages in a personal frame of mind that get read by someone in a business frame of mind.

Long-distance boyfriend sends his girlfriend an e-mail in the morning, saying, "Good morning." She's at work and doesn't respond. He later sends another message with a specific question, and she replies with an answer to the question. He responds with a hurt message about how she couldn't bother to take the time to say good morning. What their e-mails didn't convey was: "I'm at home, feeling lonely, and I miss you" and "I'm busy at work, and I know that I'll see you this weekend."

Occasionally—but not as often as most people think—the implicit message in a communication is a request for the speaker to do something. The teenage boy who says "I'm hungry" isn't just making small talk. (A teenager's appetite is not an idle thing.) Usually, however, the most important implicit message in what people say is the feeling behind the content.

When we're little, before we learn to act grown up by masking our feelings, our communications are full of ill-disguised emotion. You don't have to be a linguistics expert to figure out what a child is feeling when she says "There's monsters under my bed" or "Nobody wants to play with me." The same emotions may be implicit, if less obviously stated, when an adult says "I've got that big meeting coming up tomorrow" or "I called to see if Fred wanted to go to the movies, but he didn't call back." One of the most effective ways to improve understanding is to listen for the implicit feelings in what people say.

Much of communication is implicit and—when people are on the same wavelength—decoded automatically. Often, however, what's implicit—what we take for granted—isn't obvious to everyone. Much misunderstanding could be cleared up if we learned to do two things: appreciate the other person's perspective and clarify what remains implicit.

"Is This a Good Time?"

The context of communication is the setting: the time, the place, who else is present, and, because communication can't be reduced to the obvious, people's expectations. We ordinarily accommodate our talking and listening to the context without thinking about it. We don't spring bad news on people the minute they walk in the door, we don't talk loudly on cell phones in public, and we don't argue in front of the kids. (As you can't see by the twinkle in my eye, I'm being ironic.)

No matter how much certain people care about us, there are times when they don't have the energy and patience to listen. If a husband calls his wife at work and starts to talk at length about something that doesn't seem terribly important, she may get impatient sooner than she would if the same conversation occurred at home. By contrast, even though her husband usually retreats behind the paper at the end of the day, a wife may succeed in getting his attention by signaling her need for it. "Honey, I need to talk to you about something."

Unfortunately, in many relationships people have different preferred times to talk. He likes to talk when he comes home at the end of the day. She prefers to talk later, when they're watching TV or getting ready for bed. Fishing for understanding at the wrong time is like trying to catch a trout in the noonday sun.

• • •

When to talk: not when your partner needs some space or time to be alone.

• • •

That timing affects the listening we get may be painfully obvious; unfortunately, when needs collide, the resulting failures of understanding are obviously painful. The end of the day can be especially difficult. Partners may be frazzled. Worn out from running around all day, trying to make other people happy, attending mind-deadening meetings, fighting traffic, or chasing after children and answering endless questions, they have little energy left over for hearing each other.

The unhappy irony is that the domestic conversation people are too tired to engage in might provide just the emotional refueling they need. Talking and listening reinvigorate us. If we take listening for granted, we may assume that the people we care about will listen to us whenever we feel like talking. But good listening doesn't happen automatically. You have to find the right time to approach people.

Setting has an obvious effect on listening—in terms of privacy and noise level, for example—and an equally powerful effect in terms of conditioned cues. Familiar settings, like a therapist's office or a friend's kitchen, can be reassuring places in which to open up. Other familiar settings, like your own kitchen or bedroom, may be anything but conducive to conversation. Memories of misunderstanding and distraction cling to some places like the smell of wet dog.

Conversation in various settings is governed by unwritten rules, some of which are obvious (to most people). At cocktail parties, for example, where conversational subgroups constantly shift, conversations may be warm, candid, even intimate, but they are also brief (which may explain the warmth and candor). Anyone who tries to talk too long in a such a setting may strain a listener's sense of decorum.

Rules of decorum are based on a shared sense of what's appropriate and probably originate from practical considerations, like noninterference with others and respect for special places. Thus, talking loudly in a cathedral, on a train, or at the movies is frowned on.[4] Because rules of decorum are implicit and widely shared, we tend to take them for granted, not realizing that we have done so until we or someone else breaks them.

In addition to general rules of propriety, most of us have personal preferences for settings in which we're comfortable talking. Some people like to talk on the telephone, for example. (Why, I have no idea.) Some people like to talk when they go for a ride in the car; others prefer to read or look out the window. And, of course, we may be in the mood for conversation in a particular setting at one time and not another. Often the best way to get someone's attention is to invite him or her away from

---

[4]People who get annoyed at those who talk in the movies forget that the advent of DVD rentals has blurred the distinction between movie theater and living room. They also fail to consider situational priorities that might make theater conversation understandable. Yes, even people who talk in the movies deserve consideration, and so they should be shot as painlessly as possible.

familiar surroundings—by taking a walk, say, or going out to a restaurant. Many of these preferences are sufficiently obvious that we adjust to them automatically. We know not to call certain people at home in the evening, and we learn the most promising times and places to get the listening we need. When we don't, feelings get hurt. We blame others for not hearing us, or we feel put upon by their lack of consideration in imposing on us at the wrong time.

Whenever conversation takes place in the presence of others, some aspects of listening are accentuated while others are suppressed. If a couple goes out to dinner and the man talks about problems at work, the woman will probably listen more intently than she does at home because the setting suggests intimacy. If they bring along the children, however, she's liable to be less attentive to him and also less likely to talk about her own concerns. Sometimes that's *why* people bring the children. Togetherness is a hedge against intimacy as well as loneliness.

Most of us have had the disconcerting experience of talking to someone who seems to be interested until someone else appears. Sometimes this is unavoidable. If two people are having lunch and a third person joins them, it's not reasonable to expect to continue a private conversation. But in other instances the person talking about something important might expect the listener not to permit an interruption—to say, for example, to a telephone caller, "Sorry, I can't talk now; I'm busy." Or if two people are having a confidential conversation in a public place, one might expect the other to greet a casual acquaintance who happens by, but not to break off the conversation or encourage the third person to join in.

• • •

**Third parties are to intimate conversation
what rain is to picnics.**

• • •

Sometimes the effect of third parties works the other way. An adult may show more animated interest in a child's conversation when other adults are watching. Similarly, a man who often interrupts his wife at home may show more respect and forbearance when they're out with another couple.

I remember once when I was being interviewed on a morning television show how the host, an attractive woman in her early forties, was intrigued by the book I'd written. She sat very close, kept her eyes on mine, and asked all the right questions. Here was this radiant woman, totally engrossed in what I had to say. It was very flattering. Then a commercial break came up, and the light in her face went out like the light on the camera. I ceased to exist. After the break the interview resumed, and so did my interviewer's show of interest. Her pretense, in the face of a whole audience of third parties (and my susceptibility), was disconcerting; but after all, it was her job to show interest.

Why Some People Are So Hard to Listen To

Even when you play by the rules, some people are hard to listen to. In some cases that's because their accounts run on to Homeric length. They're generous with details. You ask about their vacation and they tell you about packing the car, getting lost on the way, and all the various wrong turns. They tell you about the weather and who said what and where they ate lunch and what they had for dinner, and they keep telling you until something other than tact stops them. Others may not talk at all about themselves but instead go on at great windy length about everyone else, all those inconsiderate others who are such problems in their lives.

It's also hard to listen to people who talk incessantly about their preoccupations—a mother with a difficult child who talks of little else, a careerist who talks constantly about his work, a man who's always complaining about his sinus trouble. One person's headache can become another's if she has to hear about it all the time. It isn't just the repetition that we tire of; it's being cast in the helpless role of one who is importuned about a problem with no solution, or at least no solution the complainer wants to consider. (If the complainer doesn't expect a solution, a simple acknowledgment of his feelings—"Gee, that's too bad"—may give a satisfactory punctuation to the exchange.)

Some people who talk too much are like that with everybody, but often, whether we appreciate it or not, some of them talk at such length with us because they talk so little with anyone else. Who other than his wife does the man with no friends talk to? Who other than the friend who seems to have her life together does the overburdened wife talk to? Some people need our attention, but if the conversation is consistently one-sided, maybe part of the reason is that we respond too passively.

Sometimes speakers are hard to listen to because they're unaware of what they've said—or of its infuriating implications. When the listener reacts to what is implied, the speaker responds with righteous indignation, wounded by the listener's "overreaction." If a mother says to her teenage daughter "Is that what you're wearing to school?" and the daughter bursts into tears and says "You're always criticizing me!" the mother might protest that the daughter is reacting unreasonably. "All I said was 'Is that what you're wearing to school?' How come you get so upset about a simple question?" Such questions are as simple as parents are free of judgment and children are free of sensitivity to it.

My father has a way of packing what feels like a whole lot of belittling into one little innocent statement that drives me crazy. If I tell him that something is so, even when it's not something particularly unusual or controversial, he'll often say "It could be." Arghh!! I think he does this because he can't tolerate overt conflict. So if you tell him something he didn't know or isn't convinced is the case, he says "It could be." To me, this feels worse than an argument. An argument, you can argue with. "It could be" makes you feel discounted. One consequence of these interchanges is that I have become stubborn in my opinions. Having had my fill of being doubted, I can't stand not to be believed when I'm stating a fact. Like the fact that Lake Champlain is one of the five Great Lakes.

In case you think I've slid from talking about speakers to complaining about listeners, you're right. While it's possible in the abstract to separate speakers and listeners, in practice they are inextricably intertwined. Listening is codetermined.

Some people are hard to listen to because they say so little, or at least little of a personal nature. If the urge to voice true feelings to sympathetic ears is such a basic human motive, why are so many people numb and silent? Because life happens to them—slights, hurts, cruelty, mockery, and shame. These things are hard on the heart.

We come to relationships wounded. Longing for attention, we don't always get it. Expecting to be taken seriously, we get argued with or ignored. Needing to share our feelings, we run into criticism or unwanted advice. Opening up and getting no response, or worse, humiliation, is like walking into a wall in the dark. If this happens often enough, we shut down and erect our own walls.

Although a speaker's reticence may be seen as a personality trait, such tendencies are really nothing more than habits based on expectations formed from past relationships.

• • •

People who don't talk to us are people who don't expect us to listen.

• • •

Therapists who encounter resistance to speaking freely engage in what is called *defense analysis*—pointing out to the patient *that* he is holding back, *how* he is holding back (perhaps by talking about trivia), and speculating about *what* might be on his mind and *why* he might hesitate to bring it up. Therapists have license that the average person lacks to ask such probing questions, but it's not against the law to inquire if a friend is finding it difficult to open up for some reason or to point out that she doesn't seem to talk much about herself. We shape our relationships by our response.

"No, Everything's Fine ... "

When you ask someone if something is wrong and the answer is a not-very-convincing "no," how do you respond? One common response is to say "You don't look fine." This may be intended as an invitation, but it doesn't come across that way. Pressing a reticent person to open up or getting annoyed at the person for not doing so presumes that he or she has no good reason for not telling you what's wrong. People don't do anything for no reason.

When someone seems reluctant to tell you what's bothering him, you might make an informed guess about why the person is reluctant to say what's on his mind. "Are you afraid of how I might respond?" If you think the person just doesn't want to get into it, you can ask "Is it something you're hesitant to talk about?" Don't push too hard, though. If someone tells you she doesn't want to talk to you about something and you keep pushing, she might decide she was right to think you can't be trusted to accept her feelings.

Does the person who isn't very forthcoming with you have reason to believe that you're interested in what he thinks and feels? That you'll listen without interrupting? That you can tolerate disagreement? Anger? Openness is a product of interaction.

Men Are from Mars?

As we head further into the twenty-first century, the social construction of gender—men do this, women do that—polarizes relations between the sexes as never before. As the old complementarity gives way to a new symmetry, conflict seems to be the price for equality.

Several books in recent years gained enormous popularity by telling us that men and women communicate differently and then explaining what those differences are. Among the most popular was John Gray's *Men Are from Mars, Women Are from Venus*, in which the author argues that men need space while women crave company. If we learn to respect the inevitable differences that crop up between two people who live together by attributing such differences to gender rather than to stubbornness or ill will, maybe that's a good thing. And if we learn not to react unsympathetically to what our partners say, that's certainly a good thing. But perhaps the most important thing is not so much learning *how* to react to these other, alien creatures, but learning not to *overreact* and learning instead to listen. Perhaps the best response to Freud's famous question "What do women want?" might have been "Why don't you ask—and then listen?"

Once, differences between men and women were thought to be bred in the bone, and this biological determinism was used to justify all manner of inequity. After years of effort to break down these separate but unequal categories, a new wave of feminist scholars reasserted what they once fought: gender differences. Jean Baker Miller emphasized responsiveness and mutuality as especially important to women in relationships,[5] and Carol Gilligan argued that for women the qualities of care and connection are fundamental to selfhood, organizers of identity, and moral development.[6] According to Gilligan, men build towers and women build webs.

Thus far the greatest impact of the new work by feminist psychologists

---

[5]Jean Baker Miller, *Toward a New Psychology of Women* (Boston: Beacon Press, 1976).

[6]Carol Gilligan, *In a Different Voice* (Cambridge, MA: Harvard University Press, 1982).

has been a reaffirmation of gender differences—but this time with a positive construction of the psychology of women. In her book, *The Reproduction of Mothering*, Nancy Chodorow pointed out that because boys and girls are parented primarily by mothers, they grow up with different orientations to attachment and independence.[7] Boys must separate themselves from their mothers to claim their masculinity, which is why boys of a certain age start shrinking from their mothers' hugs and why "sissy" and "mamma's boy" are still such powerful invectives. Girls, on the other hand, do not have to renounce their mothers' caring and connection to become women; they learn to become themselves *through* connection.

In the wake of Nancy Chodorow and Carol Gilligan, the idea of inherent gender differences has come to define the discourse on men and women to such an extent that many writers now take for granted that women are fundamentally different from men in ways that make them better at listening. For people who accept this premise, life is simple: All the complexities of relationship can be dispensed with in favor of one all-purpose explanation. Men do this; women do that. End of discussion.

This new wave of sexual typecasting is reflected in the popular reception of books that reduce every nuance, every polarity of conversation between men and women to one gender distinction: men seek power; women seek relationship. Sadly, a lot of people now take this for granted.

Perhaps the best way to begin making a difference in the quality of listening between men and women is to unmake a difference. My point isn't that there aren't conversational differences between men and women but that perhaps it's time to stop exaggerating and glorifying them.

Why are so many women and men so willing to assume that we're separated by a vast gender gap, that we speak different languages, and that our destinies take us in different directions? Is it really a woman's nature to be caring and seek connection? Is it really a man's nature to be independent and seek power? Or do these polarities reflect the ways our culture has—thus far—shaped the universal yearning to be appreciated?

Sometimes social and political factors provide the underlying explanation for so-called gender distinctions. Might caring, for example, which has been represented as a gender difference, be more adequately under-

---

[7]Nancy Chodorow, *The Reproduction of Mothering: Psychoanalysis and the Sociology of Gender* (Berkeley: University of California Press, 1978).

stood as a way of negotiating from a position of low power? Perhaps some women (and some men) are caring because of a need to please, which stems from a lack of a sense of personal power. Thus the same woman who appeals to the need for caring in debates with her husband may emphasize rules in arguments with her children. The same social embeddedness that promotes caring may sometimes make it difficult for women to recognize their own self-interest. Perhaps rather than our apologizing for or celebrating gender differences, it might be more useful for us to talk *with* each other, instead of about each other, and to move toward partnership, not polarization.

Perhaps if we started listening to one another we could move toward greater balance, in ourselves and our relationships. Perhaps women raised to believe that happiness is to be found in selfless service to others could learn more respect for their own strivings and capacity for independent achievement. Perhaps men who seek identity only in achievement could learn greater respect for the neglected dimensions of caring and concern. In the process of relaxing rigid definitions of what it means to be a man or a woman, perhaps fathers might learn to lower the walls they build around themselves and reduce the gulf across which they relate to others and guard their masculinity. Perhaps mothers, in learning more respect for their own self-interest, could develop more respect for the boundary between themselves and their children and allow the children more room to become themselves.

If we can avoid thinking of gender differences as fixed and given, perhaps we might begin to entertain the possibility that boys can identify with their mothers' nurturance and care to become more fully realized men and better fathers. Similarly, we might begin to see that girls can identify with their fathers as well as their mothers and feel entitled to be independent persons with their own agendas. Maybe God invented the idea of two parents so that children could draw on the best of both of them.

Comforting as it may be to blame lack of understanding on other people's stubbornness or insensitivity or gender, the reasons we don't listen to each other turn out to be more complex. It isn't selfishness, but complications of character and relationship that keep us from listening and being listened to.

A fuller appreciation of the dynamics of listening makes it a little easier for us to begin hearing each other. Is it necessary to dissect every misunderstanding and analyze it according to message, subtext, context, speaker, listener, and response? Of course not. The simple, heroic act of stepping back from our own injured feelings and considering the other person's point of view is quite enough of an accomplishment.

So why are we so sensitive to misunderstanding that we have trouble seeing the other person's side of things? To answer that question and continue to move toward hearing each other, let's look more closely in the next chapter at the emotional factors that complicate listening.

Quiz

To help you become more aware of your own listening habits, complete the following questionnaire. Answer the questions honestly, and because we listen differently to different people, think of a specific person you have a relationship with when you answer these questions. You might want to do this twice, once with a family member in mind and once with a coworker or friend in mind.

How Good a Listener Are You?

When someone is talking to you, do you:

1—Almost never   2—Sometimes   3—Often   4—Almost always

____   1. Make people feel that you're interested in them and what they have to say?

____   2. Think about what you want to say while others are talking?

____   3. Acknowledge what the speaker says before offering your own point of view?

____   4. Jump in before the other person has finished speaking?

____   5. Allow people to complain without arguing with them?

____   6. Offer advice before you're asked?

____   7. Concentrate on figuring out what other people are trying to say, not just respond to the words they use?

___ 8. Share similar experiences of your own rather than inviting the speaker to elaborate on his or her experience?

___ 9. Get other people to tell you a lot about themselves?

___ 10. Assume you know what someone is going to say before he or she is finished?

___ 11. Restate messages or instructions to make sure you understood correctly?

___ 12. Make judgments about who is worth listening to and who isn't?

___ 13. Make a concerted effort to focus on the speaker and understand what he or she is trying to say?

___ 14. Tune out when someone starts to ramble on, rather than trying to get involved and make the conversation more interesting?

___ 15. Accept criticism without getting defensive?

___ 16. Think of listening as instinctive, rather than as a skill that requires making an effort?

___ 17. Make an active effort to get other people to say what they think and feel about things?

___ 18. Pretend to be listening when you're not?

___ 19. Respect what other people have to say?

___ 20. Feel that listening to other people complain is annoying?

___ 21. Make effective use of questions to invite people to say what's on their minds?

___ 22. Make distracting comments when other people are talking?

___ 23. Think other people consider you to be a good listener?

___ 24. Tell people you know how they feel?

___ 25. Don't lose your cool when somebody gets angry at you?

Scoring

For the odd-numbered questions, give yourself four points for each question you answered "Almost always"; three points for "Often"; two points for "Sometimes"; and one point for "Almost never." For the even-numbered questions, the scoring is reversed: four points for "Almost never"; three for "Sometimes"; two for "Often"; and one for "Almost always." Total the number of points.

85–96 Excellent

73–84 Above average

61–72 Average

49–60 Below average

25–48 Poor

. . . .

1. If you got a high score on this questionnaire, congratulations. Read on to reinforce what you're already doing and perhaps get some additional ideas for improvement. If you scored less well, pick out one bad habit at a time and practice letting others finish talking, and then let them know what you think they're saying before you say what's on your mind. Just this will go a long way.

2. During the next few days, pick out a couple of relationships that are important to you and try to identify two or three things that get in the way of your listening. Common interferences include: being preoccupied, trying to do two things at once, having negative thoughts about the speaker ("He's always complaining"), not being interested in the topic, wanting to say something about yourself, wanting to give advice, wanting to share something similar, being judgmental.

   Once you identify two or three of your own bad listening habits, practice eliminating one of those impediments for a week, but only in conversations that you decide are important to you.

Part Two

. . .

The Real Reasons People Don't Listen

4

. . .

"When Is It My Turn?"

The Heart of Listening:
The Struggle to Suspend Our Own Needs

Forty years ago I took my first course in how to be a good listener. I was in graduate school, and the course was called Elementary Clinical Methods. We learned about making eye contact and asking open-ended questions and how to parry personal inquiries with the therapist's famous evasion, "Why do you ask?" We practiced on each other, and I learned a lot of interesting things about my classmates. Then we went to the state hospital to practice on patients, and I learned that maybe I wasn't cut out for this work.

It was the first time I'd ever been in a mental hospital, and I approached it with fascination and horror. Maybe I expected to see an axe murderer or perhaps a scene out of *The Snake Pit*. In those days before the widespread use of tranquilizers, some of the back wards *were* snake pits. But in the ward for new admissions, where they sent us, the patients were mostly just very unhappy people.

My first real patient was a young mother who'd become depressed after coming home from the hospital with her second baby. She looked disheveled and lonely, and I felt sorry for her. I asked her why she'd come to the hospital and why she felt so hopeless and where she grew up and things like that. She answered my questions, but the interview never really went anywhere. Every time I'd ask another question, she'd respond, but only briefly, and then wait for me to say something. Since I didn't have anything to say, it was an awkward wait.

It was my first interview, and I was very disappointed that it didn't go well. Eventually I learned not to ask so many questions and, if people didn't seem to have much to say, to comment on that, inviting them to explain their reticence rather than trying to fight it with questions. But the real problem in that first interview didn't have to do with technique. I wasn't really interested in that woman; I was more interested in being a therapist.

This troubling experience illustrates the most vital and difficult requirement for listening. Genuine listening demands taking an interest in the speaker and what he or she has to say.

Taking an interest can easily be sentimentalized by equating it with sincerity or caring. Sincerity and caring are certainly fine characteristics, but listening isn't a matter of character, nor is it something that nice people do automatically. To take an interest in someone else, we must suspend the interests of the self.

• • •

**Listening is the art by which we use empathy to reach
across the space between us. Passive attention doesn't work.**

• • •

Not only is listening an active process; it often takes a deliberate effort to suspend our own needs and reactions—as Roxanne's mother so bravely demonstrated by holding her own feelings in check long enough to listen to her daughter's fierce resentment. To listen well, you must hold back what you have to say and control the urge to interrupt or argue.

Kiana was enjoying going to the gym more now that she'd found a workout partner. Marilyn knew a lot about exercise and stretching and always seemed to have interesting things to say. Theirs was a nice, easy friendship, but so far it didn't extend beyond the gym.

One rainy morning, Marilyn came late and said that her basement had leaked and she had had to make an appointment with a handyman. Kiana was just about to say that she, too, had problems with leaks, but she held back her urge to talk about her own concerns to make sure Marilyn had finished.

Marilyn went from talking about her leaky basement to talking about problems she was having with her kids. Kiana really appreciated Marilyn's opening up to her and felt that their friendship had moved to a more intimate level. After their workout, Marilyn asked if Kiana and her husband would like to get together for dinner. Kiana hadn't really needed to talk about the leaks in her ceiling, and now she was glad she hadn't.

James was talking to Harry after work about starting to feel burned out. He was working long hours, losing interest in the job, and getting too little opportunity to meet new people. Harry knew exactly what James was talking about, but he suppressed the impulse to say so and continued to listen. After complaining for a while, James shifted to thinking out loud about what he could do to make life more interesting. "What I need," he said, "is something that turns me on. It doesn't have to be work. It could be getting reinvested in a hobby." By listening instead of interrupting to say "me too," Harry felt that he'd allowed James to think about doing something more than just complaining—and James's saying that he needed to rediscover something that turned him on made him realize that the same thing was missing in his life.

The act of listening requires a submersion of the self and immersion in the other. This isn't always easy. We may be interested but too concerned with instructing or reforming the other person to be truly open to his point of view. Parents have trouble hearing their children as long as they can't suspend the urge to set them straight. Even therapists, presumably exemplars of understanding, are often too busy trying to change people to really listen to them. (Unfortunately, most people aren't eager to be changed by someone who doesn't understand them.) That failures of understanding occur in psychotherapy, just as everywhere else, is a fact often missed as long as therapists remain too wrapped up in their own theories to give themselves over to sustained immersion in the other person.

Although therapists may be less likely than the average person to interrupt, some are so anxious to be perceived as sympathetic that they offer sentimentality instead of compassion. "Oh yes," they say with their eyes, "I understand how you feel." Sympathetic or not, condescending kindness from a patronizing person isn't the same thing as listening. The superficially sensitive therapist doesn't have to listen because he already knows what he wants to say: *"Oh yes, I understand."* Listening is a strenuous but silent activity.

• • •

There's a big difference between showing interest and really taking an interest.

• • •

Suspending the self does not of course mean *losing* the self—though that seems to be precisely what some people are afraid of. Otherwise, why do they insist on relentlessly repeating their own arguments, when a simple acknowledgment of what the other person says would be the first step toward mutual understanding? It's as though saying "I understand what you're trying to say" meant "You're right and I'm wrong." Or that to give someone who's angry at you a fair hearing and then say "I see why you're upset with me" meant "I surrender." Ironically, when the fear of never getting your turn is so strong that you don't hear the other person out, it becomes a self-fulfilling prophecy.

Martina was trying to explain to Zach that when she gets upset about something she just needs to talk about it without him giving her the third degree. "I never get the feeling that you're willing to just listen to me when I get upset," she said.

"Yes, but," Zach said, "if I don't understand what's bothering you, how can I help?"

"I don't necessarily need you to analyze the situation," Martina said. "Sometimes I just need you to listen to me."

"I'm happy to listen to you," Zach said, "but if I don't understand why you're upset, I don't really know what the problem is."

Can you see that both Martina and Zach are doing a good job of expressing their feelings? And that neither one is doing a very good job of listening?

I'll have some practical suggestions for breaking this pattern in Chapter 7, but first it's important to understand more about the difficulty involved in the simple art of listening.

Genuine listening involves a suspension of self. You don't always notice this because it's reflexive and taken for granted, and because in most conversations we take turns. But you might catch yourself rehearsing what you're going to say next when the other person is talking. Simply holding your tongue while someone speaks isn't the same thing as listening. To really listen you have to suspend your own agenda, forget about what you want to say, and concentrate on being a receptive vehicle for the other person.

The listener's responsiveness is experienced subjectively by the speaker as—at least temporarily—vital to a sense of being understood, of being taken seriously. Listeners feel that pressure.

The Burden of Listening

Listening puts a burden on the listener. We feel the weight of the other person's need to be heard. Attention must be paid.

But, you might object, isn't empathy a natural expression of the self? Isn't listening something we automatically extend to each other as part of being human? Yes and no. Empathy is an active form of engagement. At times we're interested in what the other person is saying, and listening is effortless. But there inevitably comes a moment when we cease to be engrossed. We lose interest or feel the urge to interrupt. It is at this moment that listening takes self-control.

• • •

Genuine listening means suspending memory, desire, and judgment—and, for a few moments at least, existing for the other person.

• • •

Suppressing the urge to talk can be harder than it sounds. After all, you have things on your mind too. To listen well, you may have to restrain yourself from disagreeing or giving advice or sharing your own experience. Temporarily, at least, listening is a one-sided relationship.

In everyday conversations, you may not notice that burden. But you can feel the pressure to be attentive whenever another person needs to talk for more than a few minutes. Even if you care about the person and are interested in what she has to say, you're caught. You need to be silent. You need to be selfless.

Doreen asked her father out to lunch so the two of them would have a chance to talk a little more personally than they did when her mother was around. But when they sat down at the restaurant, he started in on his usual diatribe against the bureaucracy. His bosses were "morons," and none of his coworkers cared about anything but "putting in their time until retirement."

Doreen had heard it all before. She nodded and looked interested and thought about her upcoming sales conference. Once or twice she started to interrupt, but something about the way her father spoke with more feeling than usual made her heart move. She stopped thinking about the sales conference and started listening to what he was saying. As she did, she began to hear the hurt and disappointment underneath his carping. Suddenly she was filled with sadness at her father's isolation. His unhappiness had less to do with his frustrations at work than that his constant complaining had made other people in the family stop listening to him. Doreen's annoyance gave way to a powerful feeling of sympathy and connection with her father. For the first time, she understood how lonely he was. Later, when she said so, her father's eyes filled with tears and he thanked her for listening.

Sometimes we're so touched by what people say that listening just happens. When your child bursts into the house and says "Guess what happened!" you don't have to work at listening.

My son was sick and stayed home yesterday, and when I called at lunchtime to ask him how he was feeling, I didn't have to make any effort to suspend my interests to tune in to his. Nor would anyone else have had to in my place. I was interested in his feelings, I intended to listen to him, and I did. We all do this dozens of times each day, at least for a few minutes.

Often, however, it's not that easy. Much of the time listening takes work.

When I came home after work, my son was lying on the couch watching TV. Again I asked how he was feeling, but this time it wasn't quite as easy for me to listen. As usual, he wasn't wearing a shirt or socks, and I had to suppress the urge to nag him about that. He was watching two brainless cartoon teenagers rating videos in which everything was either "cool" or "it sucks," and I had to make an effort to ignore that. I had things on my mind that I wanted to talk about, and I wanted to read the mail before it was time for dinner. None of these considerations was terribly pressing or unusual. It took only a little effort to suppress them long enough to listen to my son for a little while. Had he needed to talk for more than a few minutes, however, I would have had to make a more active effort to suspend these other agendas—or I would not have been able to listen.

Of course suspending your needs in order to listen means more than just allowing the other person time to talk. It doesn't mean just letting a certain amount of time elapse while that person has his say, only to leap in with your own agenda when he's finished.

We're not fooled by the feigned attentiveness of the restless narcissist, who may allow us a few minutes of airtime but is only waiting to take over the stage. On the other hand, when we open up to someone we expect to be interested and that person listens for a moment but then changes the subject to himself, we feel betrayed. It's like a slap in the face; we feel as though he didn't care about what we said.

Elena was worried about going back to get her master's degree after being out of school for six years. She'd been wanting to do this for a long time, and her friend David, who already had his degree, had encouraged her warmly. When she told him that she was concerned about doing the work, David was so enthusiastic about her finally having taken the big step that he jumped in to say how great it was that she was doing this for herself and that she'd gotten into such a good program. Elena got quiet and changed the subject. David's encouragement hadn't been very encouraging. Elena was trying to tell him that she was worried, and his saying how great it all was made her feel misunderstood. Ironically, David's expression of confidence in Elena felt like pressure, one more thing to live up to.

Like David, most people think they're better listeners than they really are. At best they allow the other person to state his case, and then they make their own interpretation of what the other person said. At worst they're preparing their own argument while the other person is still talking.

David thought he was listening but wasn't able to suspend his need to have Elena not worry or for himself to be seen as supportive long enough to hear her out. A lot of us have difficulty listening when it means having to sit still and share someone's uneasiness or uncertainty. We have to say something to make the anxiety go away.

To listen well, you have to read the needs of the speaker and respond to the context.

For example, when parents ask, "What did you do in school today?" children often say, "Nothing." What follows is an exchange of questions and monosyllabic answers. The parent wants to hear what happened in school but doesn't listen to what the child is saying. The child is saying something like "Nothing interesting enough for me to want to talk about right now. I just want to be left alone."

A child at school is exposed all day. Other kids look at you and pass judgment on what you're wearing, who you're with, what you say, how your hair is fixed, and just about anything you might do. Teachers watch to see if you did your homework and if you're paying attention and to make sure you're not making noise in the halls or generally having any fun. After being the subject of such scrutiny all day, most kids want nothing more than to be left alone. Their "nothing" isn't coy or withholding; it's self-protective.

The parents' side of this conversation isn't hard to understand either. They're curious about what goes on in their children's lives. They want to know if everything is okay. They want to know if their children are doing what they should be doing. They don't want to be shut out.

Sometimes kids say "nothing" but really do have something to say. Maybe you have to show them that you're really interested to convince them to open up. Asking them about their day and really being prepared to listen shows interest. Honoring their right to respond the way they want shows respect as well as interest—interest in them and respect for their feelings. Children who sense that their parents are interested in hearing what they have to say—as opposed to interrogating or prying—will open up when they're ready.

"What's Up?"

Questions that show awareness of the other person's interests and concerns may help reticent people open up.

Effective Questions	Ineffective Questions*
How are you coming with that project you've been working on?	How's everything?
What's been happening with your headaches lately?	How was your day?
How is your son doing in soccer?	What's new?

*Note that most ineffective conversational gambits can be answered with yes, no, or nothing.

If it's difficult to suspend the self with our children, imagine how much more difficult it is with another adult, whom we don't expect to have to indulge in any way—especially when we have our own problems.

Sometimes we fall into the habit of listening without effort because we put so much effort into other things. When we work until we're spent, we become preoccupied with our own worries and careless of concern for others. It's especially hard to listen when you feel that *you* haven't gotten the attention you need. Here's an example:

A woman who's having a bad day at the office wishes she could be at home with her five-year-old. She's envious of her college professor husband who, because it's summer, is at home all day with the boy. When she gets home, instead of complaining about her day, she asks how her husband's day went. He complains about the burden of having to amuse a five-year-old and the difficulty of figuring out what to do with all the unstructured time. She listens impatiently for a minute or two and then says, "Why are you complaining? You're lucky to have all this time off. Think of all the things you could do!" Her husband is hurt—first she asks him how his day went, then she criticizes him for telling her—and the woman herself is resentful. The woman in this example wasn't able to listen to her husband because she wasn't able to suspend her own feelings long enough to be receptive to his. After talking about this episode, the woman concluded that she needed to try harder to overcome or contain the stress of her work. (Perhaps it would be more reasonable for her to realize that when she comes home after a bad day she may need to talk about it before she's ready to listen.)

● ● ●

A good listener may need to set aside his or her own needs to tune in to the other person's, but completely selfless people don't make good listeners. You have to get listened to yourself to free you up to be receptive.

● ● ●

"But I *Am* Listening!"

The selflessness of genuine listening is hard to sustain, and so in a number of ways we fool ourselves into thinking we're listening when in fact we aren't.

"That Reminds Me of the Time ... " (Translation: "I can top that.")

When friends sit around having a casual conversation, they'll get on a particular subject and take turns telling their own stories. Carol will describe how her dachshund won't do his business outside in the winter because the minute he feels the icy snow on his paws he clickety-clicks back to the door and whines to be let in. Then Murray will tell about the time his Russian wolfhound lay at death's door for two days, until they found a small burr in his long silky fur, and when they removed it, Sasha suddenly made a miraculous recovery. Then I'll tell something fascinating (to me, at least) about my cat Ralphie's latest adventure.

In this kind of friendly exchange it's okay just to take turns. The person telling a casual anecdote doesn't need an elaborate response. However, there are times when someone has something important to say and doesn't want to hear your story until she's had a chance to finish hers—and get some acknowledgment. She needs a little time and attention. The woman who's just had her car towed away doesn't want to be interrupted to hear about the time that happened to you three years ago.

Interrupting someone to tell a similar story is a common example of how listeners don't restrain themselves. Sometimes this is annoyingly obvious, as when people draw attention to themselves by cutting in to say, "That reminds me of the time ... " Most of us don't do that when it's obvious that someone really needs to talk. If someone needs to talk, we listen. At times, however, the speaker's need for attention isn't obvious, and instead of devoting ourselves to receptive listening, we respond from our own needs. A friend starts to tell us about an accident and, in an attempt to show empathy, we interrupt to tell her about ours—which, after all, was more upsetting to us, even though it happened six months ago.

"Me Too."

"I hardly slept at all last night."

"Me, too! I was up and down all night."

When people tell stories, it's natural to be reminded of your own experience. Who do you know who frequently says "me too" when you're telling a story? When and how might such a response come across as empathy for you and make you feel understood? When does it feel like the spotlight has shifted away from you and onto the other person?

Why do people do that? Why do we interrupt to tell our own stories? Most conversation is interactive. We're engaged, and much of what people say to us triggers something in our own experience. If I tell you something annoying that my father does, you're likely to think of something annoying your father does.[1] Or if I tell you about the time I fell in love for the first time, you're likely to remember your first love. Sharing these stories may feel like an effort to establish common ground. But listening to people means hearing them out—giving them sufficient time to say what's on their mind and taking sufficient interest to follow and acknowledge their experience.

"Oh, How Awful!" (Translation: "You poor, helpless thing. What *are* we going to do?")

Another example of listeners failing to restrain themselves is responding with excessive sympathy, a gift that usually means more to the giver than the receiver. Exaggerated concern may seem less selfish than turning the conversation around to yourself, but acting distressed isn't the same thing as listening. Listening means taking in, not taking over.

Real listening requires attunement—reading and acknowledging the speaker's experience—not the kind of effusive sentiment that may fool small children but comes across to adults as patronizing and false. Expressions of concern from a person who always makes a fuss over what you say become as meaningless as Muzak.

Once again, the problem is failing to suspend the self. Instead of holding himself back long enough to listen and to hear what you're saying, the excessive responder jumps in with an expression of sympathetic concern—as if to say, "Oh, I understand ... (don't bother going on)."

---

[1] But my father is *more* annoying.

• • •

When listening is genuine, the emphasis is on the speaker, not the listener.

• • •

When something goes wrong, Christine no longer calls her mother for sympathy. She's learned that if she has the flu or one of the kids breaks a finger, not telling her mother is the only way to avoid an exaggerated show of concern. These things may not be very consequential, but she would like to share them. She doesn't, because when her mother says "Oh, that's awful!" and makes too big a deal out of everything, she feels not understood, but that her mother is worried—as though *she's* the one with the problem.

• • •

An empathic response is restrained, largely silent; following, not leading, it encourages the speaker to go deeper into his or her experience.

• • •

Part of the problem is confusing empathy with sympathy. Sympathy is more limited and limiting; it means to feel the same as rather than to be understanding. Nor does empathy mean, as many people seem to think, worrying about, praising, cheering up, gushing, consoling, or even encouraging. It means understanding.

"Well, If I Were You ... " (Translation: "Stop bothering me with your complaining and *do* something about it.")

According to some experts, men show interest by giving advice while women show interest by sharing similar experiences.[2] Unasked-for advice is annoying. It feels like being told what to do, being told that our feelings aren't valid because we wouldn't have to have them if we'd only do what the oh-so-helpful person we're talking to suggests. (Responding with a similar story, as just discussed, can be equally unwelcome, especially if the person interrupts your story before you're finished or otherwise goes on without acknowledging what you've said.) When I'm telling someone

---

[2] Deborah Tannen, *You Just Don't Understand* (New York: William Morrow, 1990).

about an experience or a problem and he or she responds with unwelcome advice, I say, "Thanks, but I don't need any advice; I just need to be listened to." (At least that's what I'd like to say.) Do men give more unasked-for advice than women do? Maybe. Not in my experience. Perhaps in yours.

A few years ago I did something uncharacteristic for me and joined a men's group. I guess I was looking for friends. It turned out to be a wonderful experience, largely because the other men in the group were all unusually interesting and thoughtful people. One day we were talking about how we respond when a friend tells us about a problem, and I was surprised to hear most of the others say that they usually try to offer advice. I thought friends didn't do that, but just listened and tried to be understanding. I guess advice-giving was trained out of me.

Of course, sometimes people *want* advice. Some individuals want advice all the time. They think other people should have an answer for their distress and should try to alleviate it. This emotional need stirs our expectations that advice is wanted. Even if it doesn't work (or get followed), giving advice may suggest that the listener takes the speaker's problems seriously.

The real issue in listening isn't whether we do or don't give advice but whether or not our response is focused on reading and responding to the other person's feelings or is simply a way of dealing with our own. Telling the person with a problem to "do something constructive" reflects a listener's inability to tolerate his or her own anxiety. So too may be pushing others to "Express your feelings" or using imperatives such as "You have to confront him about it." The difference between listening well and not is the difference between being receptive and responsive on the one hand and being reactive or introducing one's own agenda on the other. Failure to suspend the self in favor of the other reflects a lack of autonomy and a blurring of boundaries.

"Have You Heard the One about ... ?" (Translation: "Never mind what you were saying; your concerns are boring.")

Another familiar failure to restrain the self is the jokester, who's always quipping, allaying his own anxiety and calling attention to himself instead of tuning in to the speaker. There are times when your fast-quipping friend is funny and you don't mind his joking. But there are other times when you're trying to talk and his wisecracking is annoying. What the jokester offers is the thin, unreliable rhetoric of distraction in place of authentic emotional engagement. This feeling of being distracted happens a lot when you're already having a conversation with someone and the jokester joins in. Only he doesn't join in. He doesn't tune in to you and what you're saying; he just uses something you say as a trigger to make a joke.

People who joke all the time are more or less annoying, depending on how funny they are. We can understand their constant joking by realizing that they have a lot of nervous energy and may have learned to make jokes as a defense against boredom. But, like other failures to restrain the self, someone who always interrupts our conversation with gags can be annoying.

"Don't Mention It." (Translation: "I'm embarrassed about wanting to be appreciated.")

Do you remember the last time someone did you a really big favor and you were so grateful that you wanted to express your thanks in a special way? Maybe you sent flowers or gave a nice bottle of wine to show your appreciation. Or maybe you put your gratitude into words. Did the person accept your thanks or say something like "Oh, it was nothing, don't mention it"? You can understand someone's feeling embarrassed about being thanked profusely, but it leaves you feeling slightly dismissed (as if being told that your thanks weren't necessary meant that your feelings of gratitude weren't warranted). Wouldn't it be nice to be able to look someone in the eye and say "Thank you," and have him meet your eyes and say "You're welcome"?

"Don't Feel That Way." (Translation: "Don't upset me with your upset.")

You get a similar but perhaps stronger feeling of being dismissed when you tell someone about being angry or scared about something and she reassures you that there's no need to feel that way.

A lot of failed listening takes the form of telling people not to feel the way they do. It's frustrating when someone tells us we shouldn't worry or feel guilty or be so scared. The intention may be generous, but the effect is to cheat us out of having our feelings acknowledged. Most attempts to talk people out of their troubles are correctly understood as dismissive— namely, "Don't upset me with your upset."

When someone is worried or upset enough to talk about it, acknowledging those feelings is the best response. Reassuring the person that there's nothing to worry about is not responsive to him; it's responsive to the listener's own uneasiness.

If someone tells you that she's worried about the future, and you can control it, then by all means do so. Otherwise, hear her out. Even if you *know* (or think you do) that things will turn out okay (in the future), saying so (predicting the future) doesn't erase the worry (in the present). Reassuring someone instead of hearing him out may ease his mind slightly, but the disconcerting effect of not being taken seriously is usually the stronger reaction. Telling someone not to worry doesn't make her stop worrying, but it may make her stop trying to talk about her feelings to you.

The best way to keep this section simple would be to say that telling people not to feel the way they do is not listening to them and leave it at that. However, there are times when it feels okay to be reassured. You're not too happy with your new haircut, and a friend says, "No, it looks good," or you're feeling bad about not having accomplished much, and someone reminds you of all that you have accomplished and you feel better. The line between wanting to be reassured and wanting to be heard may not always be easy to discern. The more a speaker expresses self-doubt or worry or concern in a questioning or tentative way, the more likely he is to want reassurance. The stronger the feelings, the more likely he is to appreciate being heard and acknowledged. When in doubt, listen.

"Haven't We Talked about This Before?" (Translation: "Why are you still hung up about this?")

It can be hard to hear the same complaints or concerns. My advice is to blame the person talking to you for your impatience. Try not to think about the possibility that the other person keeps talking about something because you haven't ever fully acknowledged his feelings. And certainly don't consider that the annoyance you feel is related to your sense that somehow talking to you hasn't made the person feel any better. When in doubt, always blame other people for your feelings.

"Guess What?" (Translation: "Never mind what's on your mind; whatever pops into my head is bound to be more interesting.")

Jack was talking to Gail about some problems at work when Woody came over and said "Guess what?" Then he proceeded to tell them about something unrelated to what they were talking about. Had they finished? Were they interested in what he had to say? Who knows? Certainly not Woody.

If Woody's interrupting two people's conversation to talk about what was on his mind seems like such an obviously insensitive thing to do, how different is it when someone is talking to us and we change the subject without making sure the person had finished saying what he or she wanted to say?

Going Through the Motions

A good listener is someone you look forward to being around. The good listener not only pays attention to what you say but also encourages you to expand on your ideas and feelings.

• • •

However it's phrased, a good listener's response makes you feel understood and invites you to say more.

• • •

Since we always want to be seen as good listeners, we sometimes just go through the motions. We nod and say uh-huh when we're not really interested or we wait until the other person finishes even though we're not really listening to what she's saying. We all pretend to be listening occasionally, but some people make a habit of it.

Insincere listeners come in a variety of forms. Perhaps you'll recognize some of the following:

The Faker

These people feign attention. They fix their eyes intently on you when you're speaking. The intensity of their gaze reflects their concentrating on giving the impression that they're listening, rather than really listening. If you've never met one of these fake listeners (congratulations!), try meeting a politician or appearing on TV.

The Self-Conscious Listener

Self-conscious listeners want to be seen as listening but are more concerned with the appearance than the listening. They're looking at you but thinking *Am I doing okay? Do I look all right? Does the speaker think I'm intelligent?* Preoccupation with themselves gets in the way of the self-conscious listener's concentration on what you're saying.

The Amateur Therapist

Amateur therapists may be eager to play the role of listener, but they're more interested in the role than the listening. These people mistake the supporting role of listener for the leading part.

Young therapists often paraphrase everything they hear clients saying. While this sounds like a version of the acknowledgment I've said is part of good listening, it's often an attempt to pigeonhole the speaker's communication in some package of interest to the therapist—just feelings, a summary of the facts, or an analysis of some kind.

Carmen was telling her husband about the frustrations involved in arranging a conference at work. Instead of letting her explain the situation and how she felt, he kept making little judgmental summaries. "Yes, these things should have been arranged well in advance." "So, your supervisor doesn't take charge of things." "I see, there shouldn't be so many people involved in the planning process." He was probably trying to be helpful, but to Carmen his comments felt like a distraction. He was saying how he thought things should be rather than responding to her feelings about the way they were.

The problem with the amateur therapist's comments isn't failing to acknowledge what the speaker says, but doing so in a way that focuses on the listener's helpfulness rather than the speaker's feelings.

"I know what's wrong." "Here's my brilliant analysis." (Kind of like this book.)

The Active Listener

Active listening is a useful technique whereby the listener paraphrases what the speaker says. The intention is to help listeners concentrate on hearing and acknowledging what other people are saying. Unfortunately, when "active listening" gets translated into simply summing up what someone says, the focus shifts from the speaker's expression to the listener's perceptiveness.

There's nothing wrong with active listening. Acknowledging what people say is part of the essence of good listening. The problem is that when listening is reduced to a laundry list of how-tos, some people make more of an effort to show that they're listening than to actually listen. Maintaining eye contact, nodding your head, saying mm-hmm, and paraphrasing everything you hear are mechanical listening skills. They may come naturally when you're really listening, but it's important to concentrate on listening, not demonstrating it.

There's an old joke in which a depressed patient is talking to a therapist who practices active listening. The patient says "I'm depressed," and the therapist echoes "You're depressed."

The patient responds, "No, I mean it. I'm *really* depressed."

"You're *really* depressed," the therapist says.

Now exasperated, the patient says, "I'm so depressed that I feel like killing myself."

"You feel like killing yourself," says the therapist.

"I'll show you!" the patient says and then gets up, walks over to the window, and jumps out.

The therapist goes over to the window, looks out, and, after a pause, says "Plop."

Obviously, this is a parody of how paraphrasing can be a mechanical operation. The important thing isn't to summarize what someone says but to understand what he or she is feeling. So of course the therapist should have said "Ouch."

Focusing on Yourself

This little sin is what bad listening is all about. Listeners who remain focused on themselves may seem to be listening, but they're only waiting to tell their story or offer their opinion.

SPEAKER: "I hate my supervisor."

LISTENER: "Me, too. My boss is so condescending ... "

How to Overcome Focusing on Yourself

Sorry, but there are no magic answers here. The only thing to do is to concentrate on hearing the other person out. What you want to say may be perfectly legitimate, but saying it too soon skips hearing out and acknowledging what the other person was saying.

If someone says, "I hate my supervisor," and you want to say that you hate yours too, wait until it's your turn.

"I hate my supervisor."

"Gee, that's too bad. What does she do?"

Then, after that person has had a chance to elaborate, it's your turn.

But such efforts are doomed if the pressure to be heard is strong. Get the listening you need.

Do Women Listen Differently Than Men?

My assertion that the genuine listener must suspend the self runs counter to popular linguist Deborah Tannen's idea that "Many women, when they talk among themselves in situations that are casual, friendly, and focused on rapport, use cooperative overlapping: Listeners talk along with speakers to show participation and support."[3]

Yes, there are times when mutuality and the pleasures of connection are more important than the need to be heard by a self-reflecting other. But Tannen stereotypes the sexes by claiming that women engage in "rapport-talk," while men specialize in "report-talk." Men, according to Tannen, engage in self-display, while "for most women, the language of conversation is primarily the language of rapport: a way of establishing connections and negotiating relationships."[4] "For most men, talk is

---

[3] Tannen, p. 208.

[4] Tannen, p. 77.

primarily a means to preserve independence and maintain status in a hierarchical social order."[5]

Tannen gives as an example of the clashing between the sexes (which a lot of people like to think of as inevitable) a man telling a story about having to make up a shortfall in his cash register from his own pocket. The women listening to him "kept overlapping his story with comments and expressions of sympathy, elaborating on how unfair it was."[6] This, according to Tannen, is "rapport-talk." But the woman (or man) who interrupts with expressions of sympathy may not really be receptive to what you're trying to say; her frequent expressions of sympathy and elaborations may be an effort to assert herself—not in a competitive way, but as a sympathetic and appreciative person. Many "supportive" people are like that. They don't say "Look at me, I'm terrific"; they say "Look at me, I'm supportive."

When people talk about feelings—what they're excited about, what's troubling them—they want to be listened to and acknowledged, not interrupted with advice or told that someone else had a similar experience. They want listeners who will take the time to hear and acknowledge what they're saying, not turn the focus to themselves.

The inability to set aside one's own needs long enough to listen is a function of personality, state of mind, and relationship to the speaker. Some people always turn the conversation around to themselves. Narcissism or hypochondriasis or just plain immaturity leaves them with limited ability to consider anything but themselves. There are certain people who rarely talk about themselves but can't listen without imposing their own opinions on everything. These people may not be self-centered (concerned only for themselves), but they are egocentric (stuck in their own point of view) and certainly no fun to talk to.

Being listened to through the screen of a loved one's bias or anxiety leaves us feeling isolated and lonely, as though our feelings weren't valid, as though we didn't count. Children unlucky enough to grow up with biased listening become alienated from their own experience. Their view of themselves is reflected by a distorted mirror. Adults subject to egocentric listeners who aren't open to hearing their experience from their

---

[5]Tannen, p. 77.

[6]Tannen, p. 201.

perspective feel shut down, angry or deflated, and alienated from those relationships.

Those listeners who are more or less always in an unreceptive state find themselves shunned, often with no idea why. They never connect because they never cross the space between themselves and others. In Chapter 7 we'll see how listeners can learn to take in and acknowledge what people say without permeating their responses with "me" messages.

Exercises

1. Ask someone you trust to help you check your listening skills. In the course of a practice conversation, summarize what the person said after the person has completed his or her thought. By summarizing, you will become aware of how well you heard what the person was trying to communicate. What's important isn't just repeating what the person said but articulating what you think the person was trying to express.

   If you're not able to do a good job of grasping what the other person was trying to get across, try to figure out what was getting in your way. Daydreaming, forming your own response, being critical of something? Were you bored? Thinking about something else? Did you get interested in some detail of what was said and fail to concentrate on the main thing the speaker was trying to convey? These are the habits you need to overcome to become a better listener.

2. For each of the following statements from people expressing their feelings, check the response you are likely to make—not what you think you should say, but what you think you typically would say.

   a. "I've had a terrible headache all afternoon."
      (1) Maybe you should take some aspirin.
      (2) Maybe you shouldn't drink so much coffee.
      (3) Gee, that's a shame.
      (4) Gee, that's a shame. When did it start?
      (5) I've had a headache, too. Maybe it has something to do with a change in atmospheric pressure.

b. "I can't decide what to wear."

    (1) Why don't you wear—.

    (2) Nobody is going to care what you wear.

    (3) I know, it's tough to decide.

    (4) I know the feeling. What were you thinking of wearing?

    (5) I know what you mean. I can't decide what to wear either.

c. "I hardly slept at all last night."

    (1) Maybe you need to get more exercise.

    (2) You fall asleep every night in front of the TV; no wonder you have trouble sleeping.

    (3) That's too bad.

    (4) That's too bad; any idea why?

    (5) I didn't get much sleep myself last night.

d. "I hate staff meetings!"

    (1) Do you just sit there and get bored, or do you try to participate?

    (2) It's part of your job, isn't it?

    (3) Yeah, I know what you mean.

    (4) I hear that! What are yours like?

    (5) At our meetings everybody has to put in his two cents' worth.

e. "I do twice as much work as everyone else, but I don't get any recognition for it."

    (1) Maybe you should do a little less.

    (2) It's your own fault. You're always doing things for other people.

    (3) That's not fair.

    (4) How long has that been going on?

    (5) I know what you mean. I'm always the first person at work and the last to leave.

f. "I hardly made any progress on that project today. Every time I'd start to work on it, something would come up and I'd get sidetracked."

    (1) Why don't you try shutting your office door and turning off the phone?

    (2) You'll never get it done if you keep letting yourself get interrupted.

    (3) That's too bad.

    (4) You kept getting sidetracked?

    (5) I'm getting like that myself lately. Whenever I have something important to do, I seem to find so many other things to do.

In each of these examples, choice (1) is advice, (2) is criticism, (3) is an empathic comment that closes off conversation, (4) is an empathic comment that opens up conversation, and (5) is talking about yourself. Is there a pattern to the responses you typically make?

Practice making empathic comments that invite people to elaborate or go deeper with what they are saying.

5

...

"You Hear Only
What You Want to Hear"

How Hidden Assumptions
Prejudice Listening

Listening, as we've seen, takes effort. But sometimes that effort is prejudiced: Our biases filter what we hear and how we respond. Those biases take the form of preconceived expectations and defensive reactions. I'll explain how what we expect to hear filters what we do hear in this chapter and then get to emotional reactivity in the next. Understand, though, that just as it isn't always easy to separate the speaker's and listener's contributions to misunderstanding, it isn't always possible to separate assumptions from emotions that interfere with listening.

How Our Attitude about the Speaker Biases
What We Hear

One way to learn something about the forces that influence listening is to hear the same story from two different sides.

Lucy was a special-education teacher who had a humiliating encounter with the principal of her school. When the principal needed to find space for a new reading instructor, she sent Lucy a memo saying that she would have to move to a small room in the basement, previously used for storage. Lucy prided herself on being flexible, but being banished to the basement made her feel humiliated and that the principal had little respect for the special needs of her children.

When Lucy called to discuss this unsatisfactory arrangement, the principal made an appointment to see her that afternoon. But when Lucy showed up at four o'clock, the principal had gone to another meeting and left a note suggesting they get together later. Ten days went by before the principal finally made time to talk to her. By that point Lucy had to make an effort to control her anger to make the case, as calmly as possible, that moving to the basement just wasn't acceptable. Instead of listening, the principal, who'd obviously made up her mind, got defensive. At one point, when Lucy protested that the specially equipped classroom in which the children now met had always been her room, the principal said archly, "Oh, did you bring it from home?" Lucy left the meeting in tears.

As soon as she got home, Lucy called her sister, who since their mother's death was the only living member of her family. But when Lucy tried to explain what had happened, Katrine kept interrupting with questions. "What did you say that made that woman so defensive? You must have said something to set her off like that." Lucy couldn't believe it. Instead of being supportive, her sister was blaming *her* for the incident. It felt like a slap in the face. "Just listen, Katrine, will you!" she pleaded. That shut Katrine up for the moment, but Lucy could tell that her sister wasn't sympathetic and wasn't really listening, so she said good-bye and hung up.

When Lucy told me about this incident two days later, she said that her sister hadn't been there for her when she'd needed her. It certainly sounded that way. But by a strange twist of fate, I got to hear Katrine's version of the same event the following week.

According to Katrine, she's had lifelong problems talking with her sister. "Lucy has always dominated our conversations. She loves to talk about herself, but she hardly ever listens to anything I have to say. If I pause for a minute, she immediately jumps in with some comment or criticism." But what bothered Katrine most was that Lucy was always complaining. "She's always telling me about hassles with somebody—other teachers, neighbors, supermarket clerks, even the nice old man in the Chinese take-out place. And it's always the other person's fault. I used to try to listen—after all, she is my sister. But as I've gotten older, I just don't have time for her negativism." According to Katrine, Lucy was hard to listen to because she'd used up her credit.

It's not uncommon for speakers not to be heard because their credibility is low. A father's credibility, for example, may be determined by whether his wife and children think he's tuned in to what's going on in the family or too preoccupied with his work to have any idea about what's happening at home. If he's had an affair or drinks too much—even though he preaches virtuousness to the children—they may not respect him enough to hear what he has to say. A parent's status in the world also affects his or her credibility. A father who is laid off and out of work may lose credibility. This may not be because his family is judgmental, but because people who have lost self-respect in their own eyes often express themselves with a bitter edge that makes them hard to listen to. Listening is always code-termined.

The minute you pick up the phone and hear some people's voices, you're on guard. They're asking you how things are going, but you're waiting for the pitch. They call only when they want something. Even if you want to be friends, the one-sided nature of these relationships wears thin after a while. When you answer the phone and they say hello, they can probably hear the enthusiasm drop out of your voice. Do they have any idea why?

Credibility is also influenced by whether you're viewed as being in an appropriate position within a particular setting. A colleague who's seen as not really caring about what goes on at work may not be listened to even when he has something worthwhile to say. A mother who talks to her adolescent children as though they were still six years old may be experienced as out of touch and therefore incapable of having legitimate concerns.

A lot of grandparents don't get heard when they give advice about childrearing. Their mistake isn't necessarily being intrusive but rather being out of touch with their children's insecurity about being parents. The grandparents aren't heard because their children perceive their advice as undermining their own uncertain authority. In this case, the grandparents' mistake may be treating their children as though they were *more* grown up, in charge and confident, than they feel.

A speaker's credibility is also affected by whether or not his or her messages are clear and pertinent. If your father-in-law muddles his messages with malapropisms and tangential references, you may try to understand him as part of building a relationship with your spouse's family. But if you have to work too hard at it, after a while you may give up. If your father always changes the subject to talk about himself, you may get out of the habit of listening. People who abuse the privilege of our listening by going on and on or flitting from one subject to another may create the expectation that listening to them is too much work, so why bother?

When the speaker has lost credibility but the relationship has a good track record, you might pay attention even though you may not really hear. You might give the aunt who's always been nice to you the courtesy of your attention even though you don't respect her enough to really listen to what she's saying. But if there is relentless repetition of a message—any message—you're likely to withdraw even the courtesy of attention, replacing it with annoyance or distance.

If a friend can't stop talking about her ex-boyfriend, you may get tired of hearing it. And perhaps frustrated that she won't let go. The same thing happens if a friend going though a divorce can't talk about anything but what a bitch his ex is.

How Our Expectations Make Us Hypersensitive: The Discoveries of Object Relations Theory

Our relationships to each other depend on our capacity to transcend immediate experience by making a reproduction of it inside the mind, where we can then manipulate the possibilities. A simple example of this is a baby learning to tolerate his mother's absence by remembering her presence and relying on her return. This mental representation of experience can be the source of adaptive flexibility or of rigid inflexibility that sets some people at odds with the world around them.

From the start, our lives revolve around relations with others. The residue of these relationships leaves internal images of self, other, and self-in-relation-to-others. As adults we react not only to the actual other but also to an internal other. *Object relations theory* focuses on this internal other—the mental images we have of other people, built up from experience and expectation.[1]

---

[1] *Object relations* may seem a cold-blooded term for human interactions, but *objects* refer to

The details of object relations theory are rich with particulars for explaining our assumptions and emotional sensitivities, but the essence is quite simple: We relate to people in the present on the basis of expectations from the past. (A man who emerges from puppyhood with a clear picture of his father lording it over his mother may vow always to be kind and considerate to his own wife—at all times unstinting in his criticism and counsel.)

Contemporary relationships and earlier ones (encoded in the inner world of objects) interact in circular fashion. Life circumstances maintain internal expectations and are chosen because of them and interpreted in light of them.

Alice sometimes felt overwhelmed by all the people in her life who depended on her. She was the one responsible for taking care of her aging parents, even though her brother lived a lot closer than she did. Her thirty-year-old daughter called her three or four times a week to complain about something or ask for advice. Several people at work were always asking for her help on various things, even though she had her own projects to look after. What Alice forgot was that she liked doing things for people. It made her feel good. She sought out opportunities to be helpful. She grew up being rewarded for being the "good daughter" and was still playing that role, including with the two people who taught it to her in the first place.

Terry had a reasonably full life but no real friends. As a boy he had friends but never got too close to any of them. He didn't want to feel out of control or that he'd lost any of his freedom to come and go as he pleased. Beginning in college, he got more involved with what he was doing and less involved with friends. He avoided small talk because he felt it was taking him away from more important things. Slowly he got out of the habit of socializing, and eventually when he realized that he missed having friends in his life, most of the men he wanted to get close to were too busy with their jobs and families to have much time for friendship.

---

mental images of other people that are the object of our actions, not to the people themselves.

• • •

**The past is alive in memory—and it runs our lives
more than we know.**

• • •

To understand the depth of some people's hypersensitivity to making mistakes, we might turn to Melanie Klein's notion of the *depressive position*, the painful discovery that love and hurt can go together.[2] To understand other people's rage at criticism, we might consider Ronald Fairbairn's idea that the neurotic's ego is split into an *exciting ego* (leaving him longing for total love) and a *rejecting ego* (leading him to expect rejection), so that his relationships take on an "all good" or "all bad" quality and shift dramatically from one to the other.[3] To explain why some people attack and others withdraw when they get hurt, we might look to how their families responded to their narcissistic need for attention. Some people get attention for being good; in their families anger and assertiveness are beyond the pale. For others, who get attention for achievement, vulnerability and weakness may be intolerable.

What's common to these and other object-relations formulations is the idea that the neurotic person encounters others not as an equal but as a fearful child, intimidated not so much by the reality of other people as by imagined negative responses. In this respect, we're all a little neurotic.

How We Learn to Overreact

Some of the expectations we bring to conversations are built up from the history of our relationships with specific individuals. But some of what we expect to hear is part of the deep structure of our personalities, the residue of our earliest relationships. To understand listening and the dynamics of relationship it's necessary to consider not only what goes on between people but also what goes on inside them.

---

[2]Melanie Klein, "Notes on Some Schizoid Mechanisms," *International Journal of Psycho-Analysis*, 1946, *27*, 99–110.

[3]W. Ronald D. Fairbairn, *An Object-Relations Theory of the Personality* (New York: Basic Books, 1952).

● ● ●

**More than we like to realize, we continue to live
in the shadow of the families we grew up in.**

● ● ●

The sometimes vast difference between words spoken and message intended is nothing compared to the often vaster gulf between what is said and what is heard. Whenever someone seems to be responding unreasonably, it might be useful to ask: What would make that response reasonable? Once you start thinking this way—namely, that people act the way they do for a reason—you'll know something about the way they were treated by their parents.

One reason we carry sensitivities from home around with us rather than resolving them is that most of us leave home somewhere in the transition from adolescence to mature adulthood. In the busy time of our twenties, when we're making a start on love and work, we respond to our assumption that we can't really talk to our parents by distancing ourselves from them. But then, often somewhere in our thirties, we decide to close the gap and rebuild our relationship with our parents, this time on a more mature footing.

People who decide to work on their relationship with their parents often go at it with certain unfortunate expectations. They imagine themselves righting ancient wrongs like avenging angels, or waking sleeping intimacy, as though family ties, cherished, strained, or severed, could be refashioned overnight. The truth is, when you go home, you're more like one of nature's humbler creatures, and you have to keep your wits about you to avoid getting stuck on the family's emotional flypaper.

Peggy and her parents agreed on many things—the value of hard work, the need to build something for the future, the importance of family. But agreement is something children and parents can always overcome, and Peggy and her parents managed to get into shouting matches on just about every visit. Most visits would start off well. Love and news would carry them through the first couple of days, but the inevitable blowup was like a ticking time bomb, set for three days and waiting to go off.

Peggy couldn't stop wishing her parents were different. She loved them, and they loved her; she just wished they would grow up. Her mother was loud and abrasive, eager for company but always complaining, never a kind word to say about anybody. Her father was quieter, self-possessed, cool, some would say aloof. He showed his love by offering advice, whether you wanted it or not, and by repairing things around the house, whether they needed it or not. Peggy found him impossible to talk to. When she tried to tell him what was going on in her life, he never really listened.

Unlike some people, who acknowledge the turmoil they feel on family visits but don't recognize their own contribution, Peggy was willing to look at her part in the conflict with her parents. First she figured out what it was that her parents did that made her reactive. Her mother assumed the right to criticize anything and anyone, but her meanest comments were reserved for family members who acted independently. When Peggy's sister-in-law decided to start her own business, her mother said, "Who does she think she is!" She was totally unsupportive when Peggy's cousin got a divorce, even though it had been a disastrous marriage. And when another cousin decided to move out of her parents' house (she wasn't getting married), Peggy's mother said, "There's only one reason a twenty-year-old woman gets her own apartment, and I don't happen to approve of that!"

Next Peggy learned to see how her mother's negativism and intrusiveness triggered anxiety and rage in her. The fact that she'd learned to expect it made her hypersensitive. The minute her mother started in on someone, Peggy got upset, anxious, and angry at the same time. She felt she was being pressured to join her mother in mean-spiritedness, and if she resisted she felt as though she herself were under attack. She usually held her tongue, but the effort to repress her impulse to protest only put her anger under pressure, which eventually led to an eruption. The longer she held back, the more her rage would build. When she finally did blow up, her mother would get hurt and withdraw, leaving Peggy feeling helpless and despicable at the same time.

Peggy also began to see that although she rebelled against her mother's criticisms, she had incorporated her mother's habit of assuming responsibility for other people's feelings and reactions. Whereas her mother was critical and controlling, Peggy was benignly controlling—worrying excessively about her own children, always doing things for other people. The blurred boundaries between self and loved ones were the same for mother and daughter—only their way of showing it was different. The "nicer" and more "helpful" Peggy was, the more she expected there to be no walls between her and those she cared for. She felt guilty for not doing enough and repressed her anger for not getting enough. Eventually, when her children or her friends or her husband did something that made her feel shut out, she'd erupt in anger, just as she'd done with her mother. These scenes never changed anything. As you may have discovered, venting anger isn't the same as voicing feelings in a way that makes them heard. When she first consulted me about the relationship with her mother, Peggy said that she had tried everything. Her "everything" ran the gamut from A to C, appeasement to confrontation. The alternative, calmly stating her own point of view, never occurred to her, because by the time she finally responded to her mother's criticism she was too angry to be in control.

The word for unrestrained emotionalism is *childish*. The place where we learn (or don't learn) restraint is in our families. But it isn't in childhood that we overcome childishness; that isn't in the cards. As young children, we looked up to our parents. (But then we were short and looked up to everything.) Later, if they said something to incite or provoke us, we either absorbed it or cried. It was as teenagers that we began to see through our parents, stopped putting up with the exasperating things they said, and started fighting back.

Most teenagers become so reactive to their parents that they flare up at the least hint of indignity, like kindling struck by lightning. (If you've ever had a teenager in captivity, you know what I mean.) If adolescence is a time for becoming your own person, late adolescence is a time for transforming relationships with parents from a childish basis to an adult one. Unfortunately, most of us leave home in the midst of that transformation. Distance affords us the illusion that we're grown up, but for most of us who left home at eighteen or so, our relationships with our parents remain frozen in adolescent patterns.

Only one thing robs Superman of his powers: kryptonite, a piece of his home planet. A surprising number of adult men and women are similarly rendered helpless by even a brief visit with their parents. Superman becomes mortal in contact with kryptonite; mortals become teenagers in contact with their parents. We revert to childish roles when we get anxious because we never fully learn to resist parental provocation.

• • •

Our parents may be the most important unfinished business of our lives.

• • •

Our Divided Selves

We don't easily face our own shortcomings, and it's painful to confront our failures to listen. When we do, it's natural to get discouraged: "I'm a lousy listener," "I'm selfish," "I'm too controlling." Instead of thinking of ourselves in such global, negative terms, it's possible to realize that only a part of ourselves is having trouble listening. Using a little imagination to personify our parts as subpersonalities (residues of early object relations) may lead us to their source.[4]

Take, for example, a husband who finds himself shutting his ears when his wife tries to tell him that she needs more from him. With a little introspection, he might discover a part of him that feels like a little boy who expects to be reprimanded by his mother. The little boy doesn't want to hear it; his mother's criticism makes him feel scolded and controlled; he wants to be left alone. The husband can calm down his "little boy part" by realizing—really getting it—that his wife isn't his mother. She's not trying to control him. Even if she sounds critical, what she's trying to express is her loneliness and her need for him. It's not we who are afraid to listen; it's those fearful parts of us that, once triggered, reduce us to childish insecurity.

Some of our subpersonalities manifest themselves in warring inner voices that fuel those painful and tedious arguments we have with ourselves. The rival voices are normally apparent only when we're in conflict—facing a difficult decision or torn between two choices. This is when it's wise to remember that calm fosters unity; conflict fractures it. The next time you find yourself caught up in internal debate, consider the possibility that the thoughts and feelings on either side of the argument aren't just situational. Maybe those competing voices have a lot to say. Maybe they've been saying similar things to you all your life, and maybe they've been fighting those same other voices that they're fighting now. We usually

---

[4]According to Henry A. Murray, "A personality is a full congress of orators and pressure groups, of children, demagogues, Machiavellis … Caesars and Christs. … "; "What Should Psychologists Do about Psychoanalysis?," *Journal of Abnormal and Social Psychology*, 1940, 35, 160–161.

Eric Berne's transactional analysis personified Freud's superego, ego, and id as parent, adult, and child. *Transactional Analysis in Psychotherapy* (New York: Grove Press, 1961).

In literature we find Pirandello's *Six Characters in Search of an Author* and Stevenson's tortured Dr. Jekyll and Mr. Hyde.

Although many people have used the metaphor of subpersonalities, I have found the internal family systems model of Richard Schwartz particularly useful. Richard Schwartz, *Internal Family Systems Therapy* (New York: Guilford Press, 1995).

listen to one part, the one that represents the overdeveloped parts of our personalities. Here's an example:

Once or twice a year Richard takes time off from teaching at the university to spend a week by himself at a friend's house on Cape Cod. He likes to get away to spend some concentrated time writing and unwinding. But each time he goes he gets into a debate with himself about whether to spend most of his time working or relaxing. One voice says that he should concentrate on working because that's the most important thing. The other voice counters that he's always working and that this is his only chance to enjoy himself. Each time the debate is the same, and always quite frustrating. He really wants to do both, get a lot of work done and spend a few whole days swimming and fishing. But even though the debate is always hard fought, the voice that tells him to work always wins.

The people who know us can usually predict our choices, even if we still agonize over them. In Richard's case, the voice that says work always wins over the one that says play. His wife could tell you that. And she's learned, after much trial and error, that the only way for her and the children to get the attention of the part of Richard that likes to play is to reassure the part that worries about getting enough work done. She knows, for example, that he won't be able to relax on a family vacation unless he brings along some work to do in the morning. And if she tries to get him to visit her parents for the weekend, she always helps him find a little time to get some work done. She's not just thoughtful; she's smart.

Asking for Advice

A good opportunity to learn more about the opposing voices inside you is the next time you find it necessary to ask someone's advice. The need to ask is a sign that contending voices have nearly equal claim on your attention. What is the nature of those voices? Does the question of whether or not to go to an unimportant meeting symbolize a debate between the dutiful child and the rebellious one? And if you ask someone's advice, aren't you aware of what he or she will say? And do you sometimes seek out the right person to give you the answer that part of you really wants to hear?

What does all this have to do with listening? Whenever someone asks your advice or shrinks from you or gets impatient with you, it's worthwhile to think about what parts of the person might be at war with each other. It may be useful to remember these conflicting voices when you're tempted to give obvious advice—telling people to stop drinking so much, start exercising, do their homework, or quit smoking—rather than listening for what they really want from you. Can you tell these people anything they don't already know? If not, how about trying to appreciate where they're at instead of pushing them to where you think they ought to go?

Giving predictable advice to adolescents—urging them to stop doing things that aren't good for them—is a classic mistake. The voice of "no" is one that teenagers are already well aware of. A more effective way to get through to them (or anyone else with self-destructive habits) is to adopt a more neutral attitude and simply ask them about the effects of whatever they're doing. Unfortunately, when this question comes from someone who is in fact anxious to make them change, it won't be heard. Teenagers can smell manipulation a mile away.

The compulsion to pursue self-destructive behavior isn't easily overcome with platitudinous advice. Not only do smoking and drinking and overeating feel good, but they're also supported by an inner voice that whispers, *"Go on, you deserve it!"* Sometimes our inner voices work as a team in a control-and-release cycle. The voice of self-reproach heaps on the punishment that produces the control that eventually leads to another rebellious release.

Psychologists call the interface between the voice that says "do it" and the one that says "no" the *vertical split*.[5] Unlike the horizontal split (repression), the vertical split doesn't keep wishes out of consciousness, only on the back burner. In the case of a woman who spends too much money on clothes or drinks too much, the voice on the "do it" side of the vertical split is the one that usually doesn't get heard—no one says to her "You're special; you deserve to be treated well"—and that's why she acts out its dictates. It takes empathy to bring out and reassure the shy voice that says to her, *Go ahead, you need this; you deserve it.*

Thinking in terms of subpersonalities can be especially helpful in heated discussions. Instead of thinking of being at odds with someone, it's

---

[5]Heinz Kohut, *The Analysis of the Self* (New York: International Universities Press, 1971).

more useful to think of parts of one of you trying to change parts of the other. In a typical scene provoked by a teenager's coming home late, his father gets mad and demands to know what happened. His accusatory tone makes the boy feel attacked, and he counters angrily, which drives up the father's rage to the point where his wife tells him to calm down and stop shouting. This infuriates the father, and he leaves the house. If you were the father, you would probably think of the boy as disrespectful and the mother as interfering. If you were the boy, you'd view the father as controlling. Instead, think of the conflict as being waged among parts of them. A rebellious part of the boy activates a controlling part of the father, which in turn mobilizes a protective part of the mother to shield the boy from his father's temper. If you were any one of these people and you began to think this way, how difficult would it be to control your part? How might the problem be affected if any of you could stay calm and avoid letting your reactive parts take over?

Take another example. Does the question of whether or not to confront your partner with something that's bothering you represent the competing voices of a compliant child who believes that she shouldn't complain or people will get mad at her; a hurt part; and an angry part? Of the last two, which one is more afraid to speak up? Why? If you can identify those parts that have trouble speaking up, can you find a way to reassure them? Would it help to tell the person you have trouble speaking up to about the scared part of you? Would he (or she) be more understanding if you asked for his (or her) help to express this part of you?

Let's take a look at a familiar interaction between intimate partners, using the notion of subpersonalities. A woman has trouble listening to her husband because he expresses himself in the form of tirades. Is this the sensitive and vulnerable man she married that she hears, or is it an echo of mounting anxiety and danger from long ago? And who is the "she" who's doing the hearing? The part of her who's strong and cares deeply about her husband or a little girl part who trembled to hear her parents quarreling over her father's explosive temper and her mother's shame about it in front of others?

Finding the "parts" (obstacles or constraints) that get in the way of our receptivity and then releasing these constraints is a very different way of thinking from accusing ourselves of being immature or selfish or inadequate. It isn't that we're bad listeners; it's our hidden emotional agendas that crowd out understanding and concern. When we clear away automatic emotional reactions—criticism, fear, hurt—we get to compassion, curiosity, and tenderness. Instead of condemning ourselves for being "bad listeners," we can learn to identify and relax those parts of ourselves that interfere. In so doing, we release ourselves for effective listening.

Exercises

1. Pick three people you see regularly. Write down what you generally expect them to say to you. Then write how you usually respond. How could you set aside those expectations to have a more in-depth conversation the next time you see one of those people?

   The most satisfying conversations with people we care about involve talking about our personal concerns and both getting a turn. If your conversations with someone are usually about things you care less about—the weather, the news, third parties—ask more direct questions about what you'd prefer to talk about. When it's your turn, use an orienting comment—like "There's something going on with me" or "I'd like to tell you about ... "

2. What did each of your parents do to make you feel they weren't really listening to you? How do those experiences affect how you approach conversations now?

3. How could you approach either of your parents in some completely different way the next time you're in touch with them? What makes you afraid to try doing so?

4. Try to identify and personify the defensive parts (fearful, angry, hurt) that interfere with listening in the following examples.

   a. Ivan's boss is describing how they should handle a particular project, but Ivan doesn't hear any of the details because he thinks the boss's whole approach is wrong.

   b. Monica and Charlotte are eating lunch in a Chinese restaurant. Charlotte is talking, but Monica can't stop thinking about how annoying it is that the man in the next booth is talking so loudly on his cell phone.

c. "Can I talk to you about something, honey?" Toni asks. "Not now, I'm busy," Rob says.

d. Lorraine starts telling her father about a project she's working on when he interrupts to talk about something else. Lorraine doesn't say anything, but she doesn't hear a word he says.

e. You want to tell someone how much he or she means to you, but you're afraid that kind of intimacy might make both of you feel awkward.

f. Bev is explaining to Michael what kind of toaster she wants him to exchange for the one he brought home. Michael, who doesn't have the receipt, wishes she wouldn't make such a fuss about the toaster in the first place. When he gets to the store, he can't remember what kind of toaster he's supposed to buy.

g. Mindy's father is explaining where he keeps all his important papers and what Mindy will need to take care of after he dies. She knows these things are important, but her father is still in good health, so she doesn't really pay attention to what he's saying.

h. Sharon thinks that she and Carlo should go to couples counseling, but she's afraid to bring it up for fear of how he will react.

Do you find it hard to identify the parts of these people that interfere with listening without knowing more about the people's backgrounds? The point of the exercise isn't to get the "right" answer, but to get you thinking about what kinds of things might be behind your and other people's problems in listening.

6

...

"Why Do You Always Overreact?!"

How Emotionality Makes Us Defensive

One of the reasons people don't listen is that they become emotionally reactive. Something in the speaker's message triggers hurt or anger, which provokes defensiveness and short-circuits understanding. Emotional reactivity is like throwing a switch and having the electricity come on, only instead of music you get static. The static is anxiety.

"What's *Really* Bothering You?"

The hardest messages for us to listen to without reacting emotionally are those that involve criticism. Most of us like to think that we can accept constructive criticism, and, on the other hand, most of us know people who can't.

Once a month the Outpatient Psychiatry staff at Briarcliff Medical Center reviews patient charts to assess the treatment being provided at the clinic. This may sound like a good idea, but the review has become progressively more tedious as the need to monitor bureaucratic forms has crowded out time for considering the quality of care patients are receiving.

111

At the last meeting the staff discovered that a few of the charts selected for review had already been examined at the previous month's meeting. When the director mentioned this to the secretary, she said, "Then get them yourself—I can't do everything!" and stormed out of the room.

If you believed that this kind of reaction was common from this woman, you'd have no trouble recognizing her as one of those hypersensitive people who can't take criticism. If, on the other hand, you knew her to be a very even-tempered person, you'd assume she was having a bad day. You'd be right. Her assistant was out sick and she'd had to stay three hours late the night before and come to work two hours early to get the charts ready. Of course she was on edge.

When people overreact uncharacteristically, we usually assume that something's bothering them. If our relationship with them has a history of goodwill, we give them the benefit of the doubt and try to find out what the problem is. But what about those people who regularly respond inappropriately? Are they having a bad life?

Corinne was a highly intelligent woman who couldn't allow herself to make mistakes. She kept up with *Forbes*, *Barron's*, and *The Wall Street Journal*, but she also watched ESPN and read *Sporting News*. She especially loved baseball and took pleasure in writing a newsletter about her favorite team, the Atlanta Braves, and circulating it at the office. When the team's star pitcher injured his shoulder, Corinne wrote that this might turn out to be a blessing in disguise if it allowed a certain relief pitcher to prove that he would make a good starter as some insiders suspected. When Corinne read a draft of the piece over the phone to her cousin Drew, he said it was great, except for one thing: the pitcher was injured playing against Pittsburgh, not Philadelphia, as Corinne had written. Glad to get the facts straight, Corinne corrected the error. When the newsletter came out, a senior staff member told Corinne that he loved her article, but it was Philadelphia, not Pittsburgh, where the fateful injury took place.

Corinne was so humiliated by this minor mistake that she was thrown into a tailspin. She cried and felt like a fool and couldn't bring herself to go to work the next day.

She was a shy person who preferred to express herself in writing rather than conversation; to her, being listened to meant having what she wrote appreciated. Being wrong made her feel humiliated. Instead of getting angry at her cousin for giving her the wrong information, she was ashamed of herself for not getting the story straight. Nobody likes to make mistakes, but clearly Corinne's reaction was excessive.

Another example of reacting inappropriately may be more familiar, in form if not intensity. Lenny was a devoted husband and a good provider. He did his share of household chores and was emotionally involved in the life of the family. His wife's one complaint was that he was too critical.

The only thing that struck me as unusual about this situation was the degree to which Sheila absorbed Lenny's complaints without answering with any complaints of her own. It was as if he was the lord and master, and it was her job to cater to him. When Lenny said, "You should clean all the snow off the car before you start to drive," Sheila protested feebly, "I was in a hurry to get to the cleaners." When Lenny countered, "You're always in too much of a hurry," Sheila capitulated, "I guess you're right."

Experience has taught me to listen not only to what people say but also for what they're not saying. I soon found out why Sheila hesitated to protest. One time she said, "Don't you think you're being a little unfair?" and Lenny flew into a rage. He started shouting at her. "You *never* listen to anything I say! You have *no* respect for me. You say you love me, but it's a *goddamned* lie!"

It was awful. I don't really remember all of what he said because, frankly, I was too upset. What's more, the same thing happened every time Sheila said anything critical to Lenny. His reaction was so extreme that it was impossible to really understand what he was saying.

Having read these two accounts, you can probably guess something of what both Corinne and Lenny felt. But clearly the intensity of their reactions was inappropriate to the situation. Let me also tell you that these are two instances when it's a lot easier to read about something than to witness it firsthand. Corinne's abject remorse and Lenny's rage made listening to them almost impossible. What makes people respond so inappropriately? Long memories.

From these brief descriptions, some people might say that Corinne was insecure and Lenny suffered from unresolved aggression. Others might say that Corinne's turning her anger inward and Lenny's lashing out were typical of their genders. In fact, these inferences are so general and judgmental as to constitute virtually meaningless clichés. For a more subtle appreciation of a person's overreaction you need to know its trigger.

• • •

**A listener's emotional reaction seems inappropriate
only as long as you can't see his or her memory.**

• • •

As a therapist, when I see someone responding "inappropriately," I ask myself what circumstances *would* make the response appropriate. (In my own relationships I just get upset like you do.) What would make it reasonable for a woman to feel hopelessly worthless for having made a minor mistake? (Hint: Most of us manage to survive childhood, but not all of us outgrow it.)

Corinne was the last of four children in a talented and ambitious family. She had three older brothers "who were jealous and competitive" and "never liked me." Her father was cerebral and distant; her mother was a depressed underachiever who drank too much. Corinne was the baby, but rather than being doted on she was ignored. Early on, she decided that the only possibility of ever being loved was to be the perfect child, docile and mediocre—docile so as not to burden her parents, mediocre so as not to challenge her brothers. They tolerated her as long as she played the good little sister, but they couldn't acknowledge any sign of accomplishment from her. Deprived of acceptance themselves, they belittled their little sister's achievements and mocked her mistakes. They called her "lardass," "Miss Piggy," "stupid," and "retard." Even the smallest slipup could trigger their scornful laughter. Years later Corinne was still so hypersensitive to humiliation that she sank into despair whenever she made the slightest error. The man who pointed out her mistake did not say "retard," but that's what she heard.

• • •

**When you're a little child, it's hard to fight back.
When you're an adult made to feel little, it's hard—
but not impossible.**

• • •

What made Lenny so critical of others and yet unable to tolerate criticism in return? Not the kind of cruel treatment you might expect. Lenny's parents were decent, loving people. But their lack of involvement outside the family led them to expect a lot from each other and from their children. When they didn't get what they wanted, they criticized and complained. This alone might not have made Lenny so unable to tolerate criticism. But his parents, for all their basic goodness, never gave him the empathy that would have solidified his sense of worth. Without a store of loving memories, without a sense of being taken seriously and appreciated just for himself, and without expectations of more understanding to come, Lenny harbored deep and ugly fears of worthlessness. Hard work and family devotion kept these feelings at bay, until, that is, someone said anything remotely resembling what Lenny himself feared in his heart of hearts—that he was no good.

I once had a gray-and-white cat named Tina who was perfectly friendly, except that once in a while she'd lash out violently with her claws. These attacks were totally unprovoked. One minute Tina would be purring to have her head stroked; the next minute you'd have a bloody scratch on the back of your hand. Eventually we took her to the vet and learned that she had an injured hip—possibly from a car accident when she was a kitten—so that what seemed to us like a harmless touch could actually be quite painful.

Shame and insecurity are the wounds that make people react violently to criticism. Some people retreat from hurt feelings, others attack. The most shame-sensitive individuals flare up at the slightest sign of criticism. Such people are hard to live with. But reacting to criticism with hurt and anger is something we all do. What varies is only the threshold of response.

The universal vulnerability to criticism is related to the universal yearning for love and approval. What we really want to hear is that we're terrific (sometimes "okay" will do).

Our sensitivity to criticism varies with the situation. We're hurt most by criticism of something that feels like an important part of ourselves— our motives, for example, or the products of our creativity, or, during adolescence (and sometimes slightly beyond), our appearance. We're especially sensitive to criticism from someone whose opinion we care about. The right person saying the wrong thing can puncture your ego like a pin bursting a balloon.

How to Listen to Complaints

Do you often find yourself interrupting someone who's criticizing you before the person has a chance to finish? This understandable but counterproductive impulse robs the other person of a sense of having been heard. You don't have to agree to hear what someone has to say.

To avoid getting defensive, concentrate on listening to the entire complaint. Then ask, without sarcasm, "Is there anything else?" Finally, offer your understanding of what the person was trying to say—*not a paraphrase* but what you think the other person was trying to get at.

Why Do People Complain to Us?

Behind every complaint is a request. Listen for the request and then ask if that's what the person would like.

Respond to the request by accepting it or making a counteroffer—in the spirit of trying to give the other person what he or she is asking for.

What Makes Us Intolerant?

When you're trying to figure out why you or anyone else overreacts, keep in mind one of the great ironies of understanding: We're likely to be as accepting of others as we are of ourselves. That's why those lucky enough to be raised with self-respect make better listeners. Still, you needn't be stuck where you find yourself. If you learn to respect other people's feelings, you will learn to treat your own feelings more kindly in the process.

• • •

**What we can't tolerate in others
is what we can't tolerate in ourselves.**

• • •

We can't listen well to other people as long as we project the mistaken idea that parts of us aren't good enough to be loved, respected, and treated fairly. A wider respect for human dignity flows from and enhances respect for ourselves. Tolerance and appreciation of our own and other people's feelings helps us hear and understand the hurt that inevitably lies behind anger and resentment. When our feelings aren't heard, our spirits are suppressed and distorted.

What Turns Conversations into Arguments?

Reacting emotionally to what other people say is the number-one reason conversations turn into arguments.

If you're not sure what emotional reactivity is, take inventory of your feelings the next time you rush out of the bathroom to catch the phone on the last ring—and it turns out to be somebody selling something. That agitation, that anxious upset that makes you want to slam down the phone, is emotional reactivity. Is it wrong or unjustified? No, of course not. But it's that feeling, in relationships that do count, that makes it hard to listen, hard to think straight, and hard to say what you want to say.

Reactivity is like a child interrupting an adult conversation—it isn't bad; it's inopportune. Our intrusive emotions may need to be hushed, but they may also need to be listened to later. Why are we reactive? What are the reactive parts of ourselves, and what are they reacting to? Disruptive feelings are messages from our inner spirit about something we need to change or pay attention to in our lives. Our reactivity can lead us to parts of ourselves that we haven't yet befriended—angry and resentful parts, frightened and lonely parts.

If Corinne were to tell a friend how stupid she felt for screwing up the newsletter, the friend might try to reassure her by telling her not to worry. Everyone makes mistakes. Yes, but when Corinne made a mistake, she could hear the savage brothers sneering: "Lardass! Retard!" And she'd feel again what she'd spent her whole adult life running away from: that she was ugly and stupid, nobody loved her, and nobody would ever love her.

Lenny's dishing out but not being able to take criticism might seem less unreasonable if you realized that deep down he, too, felt worthless and inconsequential. Inside him were dark and ugly voices he anxiously shut his ears to lest he get in touch with the part of him that still felt like a little boy who was never good enough.

What turns conversations into arguments for some people (not infrequently mothers) isn't so much something inside of them as the fact that they can't tolerate certain things in people close to them.

One of my patients doesn't want to hear what's going on in her daughter's life. It's too upsetting. Allison was arrested for prostitution at age fifteen. Despite her mother's heroic efforts, Allison continued to get into trouble, using drugs, hanging around with a motorcycle gang, coming home drunk night after night. Finally, when Allison was eighteen, her parents insisted that she get her own apartment. They supported her for a while, then gradually stopped paying her expenses. Allison now works as a cocktail waitress, when she works, but her parents are reasonably sure that she's using drugs and that she probably still prostitutes herself from time to time. They know she occasionally gets arrested for drunk and disorderly behavior, because they've had to go to the jail in the middle of the night to bail her out. Her mother still loves her but finds it necessary to cushion their relationship by visiting infrequently and avoiding the details of her daughter's activities, which she finds too upsetting to listen to.

This mother's avoidance is based on a correct assessment of her own vulnerability. It isn't just worry that she's avoiding; she can't listen to her daughter's troubles without feeling the need to reform her. The temptation to tell her daughter to stop taking drugs and hanging around dangerous characters (as though these were novel ideas) interferes with listening; yielding to that temptation triggers shouting matches.

The worst thing about reactivity is that it's contagious. When anxiety jumps the gap from speaker to listener, it escalates in a series of actions and reactions, which may eventually lead to an emotional cutoff. The cutoff may be as simple—and simply frustrating—as walking out of the room or as sad as someone walking out of another's life.

The next time you have the misfortune to witness two people arguing without hearing each other, notice what each of them does to keep the argument going. (If you're one of the parties to the argument, just notice what the other person does; the alternative is too demanding.) Notice how the argument could end if either one of them would let go. In the runaway logic of arguing, both parties feel compelled to get in the last word.

• • •

The world is divided into people who think they are right.

• • •

The ability to listen rests on how successfully we resist the impulse to react emotionally to the position of the other. The more actions we feel compelled to take to reduce or avoid our anxiety, the less flexible we are in relationships.

Let me give you an example from the wide perspective of a public situation—before focusing on the more anxiety-arousing settings of personal exchange. The next time you attend a lecture or observe a news conference, notice the hostile questions. You'll note that many "questions" aren't really questions at all, but rhetorical attempts to prove that the speaker is wrong and the listener is right. Observe how the speaker handles these questions. Some speakers try to remain calm by finding something to agree with; others get defensive and counterattack.

A speaker is likely to get defensive if she feels that the questioner is trying to make her wrong and himself right. "Excuse me, but haven't you overlooked ... [you dummy]?" Few such "listeners" really want answers to their questions; they just want to be right. The speaker who gets defensive and tries to counter (put down, really) the questioner often hopes to "win" the exchange by saying "No, actually ... [I am right; *you're* wrong]." In rare instances a clever speaker can succeed in putting down a hostile questioner with superior intellect or knowledge of the subject. More often the questioner, who maybe wanted to make a point, feels dismissed, cheated out of the opportunity to have his voice heard.

● ● ●

When neither party to an exchange is willing to break the spiral of reactivity, both are likely to end up feeling angry and misunderstood.

● ● ●

How to Alleviate Arguments

I don't know about you, but I hate arguments. Why do some people always have to say the opposite of whatever we say? In the interests of understanding, I've made a list of reasons people argue with us.

- **They have bad memories.** "My wife and I argue all the time about whether one of us said something or not. I wish I could record our conversations. I should know what I said, shouldn't I?"
- **They're selfish.** "My boyfriend insists that we spend Christ-

mas with his parents. Why can't we spend Christmas with my family?"

- **They're ignorant.** "We interviewed three job candidates last week, and I thought one of them was clearly the best. So it was a shock when two thirds of the group voted for one of the other candidates."

- **They're old-fashioned.** "My father doesn't have voice mail. So I often have to call several times just to give him a simple message. When I suggest that he get an answering machine he says 'What do I need one of those for?'"

- **They're stubborn.** "My wife says we should keep the car for another year before buying a new one. When I remind her that a new car will cost less now than next year, she insists that it will be cheaper in the long run to keep our present car for another twenty-five thousand miles."

- **They're naïve.** "My daughter wants to study creative writing in college. She has no idea how hard it is to make a living as a writer."

- **They're emotional.** "When I tell my boyfriend that it's too expensive to visit each other every single weekend, he gets all hurt and angry."

- **They're bossy.** "My husband insists on going out to dinner almost every night. Why can't we eat at home once in a while?"

- **They don't really listen to what we're saying.** "Whenever I bring up some chore that my boyfriend doesn't like doing and say that we don't have to do it right away, he never hears the don't, and he's always getting needlessly upset."

It's easy to see what these explanations have in common: They underscore the basic fact that when other people argue with us, it's their fault. Naturally, it's our responsibility to straighten them out.

Why, some of you sticklers for fairness might be thinking, is it never we who are selfish, stubborn, or naïve? Because what we say makes sense.

There are, of course, two sides to every argument. But when we argue, we insist on repeating our side without listening to the other person's position.

Responsive listening is a technique designed to reduce arguments by hearing the other person's side of the story before giving your own. Responsive listening allows you to shift from an adversarial stance, reflexively countering what someone else is saying, to a receptive stance, allowing the other person to express his feelings, while you put your feelings on hold. Responsive listening was developed to resolve arguments. However, as you'll see in subsequent chapters, responsive listening will enable you to improve your listening in almost any situation.

Here's how responsive listening works.

Responsive Listening

1. At the first sign of an argument, check the impulse to argue back and concentrate on listening to the other person's side of the story.

2. Invite the other person's thoughts, feelings, and wishes—without defending or disagreeing.

3. Repeat the other person's position in your own words to show what you think he or she is thinking and feeling.

4. Ask the other person to correct your impression or elaborate on his or her point of view.

5. Reserve your own response until later. On important or contentious issues, wait a day or so before giving your side of the issue. On minor matters pause and ask if the other person would be willing to hear what you think.

When someone starts to argue with what you've said, your first impulse is to explain or restate your ideas. But when two people insist on talking, neither one is likely to listen.

To break that pattern before the argument escalates, remind yourself that you're going to draw out the other person's feelings before responding with your own. Don't even start to argue; stay in control by listening.

• • •

Arguments are like ping-pong games:
It takes two to keep them going.

• • •

To really hear another person's concerns, you have to suspend your own agenda, at least temporarily. It isn't possible to listen effectively when you're just waiting to respond. It may take some effort, but the active decision to postpone responding to explore the other person's thinking is the first step in breaking the chain of argumentation.

> "I don't remember saying that, but you may be right. What do you want to do about this situation?"

• • •

**When is an argument not an argument?
When you don't argue back.**

• • •

Because most people expect arguments to focus on the outcome, it may take a little time for people to learn that you really are interested in understanding their feelings. On the first few occasions you try responsive listening, the other person may be impatient to get to a resolution. The ability to resist being drawn too quickly into making a decision begins with a conscious decision to focus first on the other person's feelings.

> "Do we have to go out to dinner every night?"
> "Why don't you like going out to dinner, honey?"

One reason people doubt that we understand how they feel is that we fail to let them know we heard them. Silence is ambiguous. Repeating the other person's position in your own words is the best way to let him know that you understand. Don't sum up what you've heard as though that should be the end of it, however, but rather as a means of inviting the other person to elaborate so that you can *really* understand.

> "Let me see if I understand. You don't like going out to dinner every night because none of the places we go to serves vegetables, and you don't feel like we're eating healthy enough?"

Notice how this paraphrase is expressed with a question. The point isn't to convey that you understand but to convey that you're trying to.

The fourth step of responsive listening is tied directly to the third. I list it separately to emphasize the importance of getting the other person to elaborate on his or her position. The point of responsive listening isn't to reach some conclusion—or to cut off the discussion—but to allow the person you're talking to tell her side of the story—and to feel that you're listening to it. The longer the other person talks, the longer the cycle of arguing is avoided. The goal is communication.

"I think I understand what you're saying, but I want to be sure. Do you mean ... ?"

"I'm not completely sure I understand what you mean. You're saying _____, but I wish you'd say more about [your position] so I can get it straight."

Sometimes, after showing that you understand the other person's reasons for not agreeing with you, you may simply want to reaffirm your position. The conversation now switches from understanding to reaching a decision. At this point, any attempt to justify your position as anything other than your personal opinion or preference only invites further debate. Just say "Well, this is how I feel," and then if a decision is required, the two of you can negotiate an agreement that hopefully takes both of your preferences into account. I'll have more to say about negotiating later.

As often as possible, it's a good idea to separate the conversation in which you try to be understanding from the one in which you have to reach a decision. Doing so makes the other person feel that you are considering his or her position, and it gives you time to review your options with less pressure. Responsive listening isn't magic. It doesn't eliminate differences of opinion. It's only a device to reduce the argumentativeness of disagreements. But you'll find that it is a very useful device—if you remember that the goal is to draw the other person out and really listen.

There are a variety of other approaches that encourage listeners to acknowledge the speaker's feelings, but most of them are designed to bring the conversation to a quick conclusion.

"I understand how you feel, but now I want to tell you what I think."

This "yes, but" approach doesn't work very well. Responsive listening is designed not to summarize conversations but to open them up. Even if your only goal is to get the other person to accept your position, getting him to talk at length about his point of view is the best way to put him in a receptive frame of mind. A perfunctory acknowledgment of feelings usually doesn't work.

When you're trying to empathize with someone's feelings, saying "I understand" isn't very understanding. It implies that you already know what the other person is trying to say. Since you already know what she's feeling, there's no need for her to talk about it.

Imagine how you'd feel if you were worried about an upcoming presentation at work, and you said to your mate something like, "Honey, you know I'm a little worried about how I'm going to handle that project I've been working on," and he responded with a perfunctory expression of sympathy, "Yeah, I know what you mean," and then turned back to what he was doing. How would you feel?

Actually, a more useful thing to say when trying to appreciate what someone is feeling is "I *don't* understand."

> "I'm not sure I really understand how you feel. Can you explain it to me?"

> "I think I understand how you feel, but I'm not certain. Can you tell me?"

• • •

The difference between saying "I'm not sure how you feel" and "I know how you feel" is the difference between showing an interest in listening and not.

• • •

The point of responsive listening isn't to get to the point where you can paraphrase what the other person has said. The point is to get that person to talk. It's the talking—the communicative act of expressing feelings to someone who cares enough to listen, not the accuracy of the listener's perception—that makes people feel understood. When it's genuine, responsive listening is a way around arguments, and a way inside other people's feelings.

Listening with a Clenched Mind

Listeners anxious to avoid conflict may not listen because they're too busy protecting themselves to be open to what someone else is trying to say. Listeners intent on talking speakers out of unhappy feelings or independent inclinations won't hear what others think because it might be threatening. Even speakers who have something worthwhile to say may not get heard if they make the other person feel criticized or misunderstood; the listener is likely to become defensive or angry and counterattack or withdraw, making listening the last thing on his or her mind. Misunderstanding is perpetuated when each one broods over the awful things the other one does and one or both of them eventually finds someone else to complain to.

Subjects Too Hot to Handle

Married couples famously have trouble talking about money, sex, and children. The problem with these subjects isn't differences of opinion but the emotional reactions those differences trigger. Even though both partners might be equally reactive, they may show it in different ways. One may press for more reasoned analysis, while the other may feel shushed and press for more emotional honesty. Each is sensitive to slights, hurts, and criticism. Some people's radar is so good that they pick up these signals even before they're sent.

After Don and Shannon have a blowup, he becomes distant. After a while, he calms down and tries to make amends. He says he's sorry for what he said. But she never apologizes. She either accepts his apology or, if she's really mad, takes it as permission to say more about what he did that upset her. Don's least favorite version of this is "You *always* do that, and I hate it!"

Finally, Don told Shannon that he truly was sorry when they argued and often could see his part in it, but it really bothered him that she never apologized. "It's like everything is my fault, like you don't have any role in our problems. It's not fair."

Shannon blew up. "What am I supposed to say, 'It's *my* fault you're so grouchy'? 'I'm sorry *you* don't like my driving'? 'I'm sorry the baby was sick'?" At this Don threw up his hands and walked out of the room.

What makes it so hard for some people to apologize? Guilty consciences. In her heart of hearts, Shannon blamed herself for everything that went wrong in their relationship. She blamed herself for Don's moods (if she was *really* a good wife, he'd be happy); she blamed herself for not enjoying sex with him more (she must be inhibited); she even blamed herself when the baby got sick (if she were a better mother, nothing bad would ever happen to her child). She came from a family that specialized in blaming. The result was extreme sensitivity to anything anyone might say that triggered her own inner self-blame. That's the nature of reactivity.

• • •

**We're most reactive to the things
we secretly accuse ourselves of.**

• • •

"How Come You Listen to Everybody But Me?"

Husbands and wives often complain that their mates never listen to their ideas but come home and announce that they just heard something very interesting—and that something is precisely what their partner has already told them. Recently, for example, when Marilyn told her husband that she'd decided to see a friend's chiropractor about her back, he hit the ceiling: "I've been telling you to see a chiropractor for years! Now all of a sudden when your precious friend Mary Elizabeth tells you, you listen. How come you never listen to me?"

Marilyn was taken aback by her husband's outburst. But even if she'd known what to say, her husband didn't stick around to hear it. He stormed out and slammed the door. Later, she did answer him at length, in her head, where most of us make our best comebacks.

True, he *had* told her to see a chiropractor. But she hadn't asked his advice. When she complained to him about her back, she wanted sympathy, not advice. He was always telling her what to do. Why couldn't he just listen?

When Marilyn told me about this episode, I thought her assertion that she wanted sympathy, not advice, from her husband was true as far as it went, but that it was missing something. It turned out that when her husband gave advice, it was usually in an intense, pressured way—his response to the anxiety her complaints generated in him. She usually ignored his advice, not just because she wasn't in the market for advice but because it was delivered with an emotional pressure that made her defensive.

This is typical of how messages get deflected. It isn't the content that makes people deaf; it's the pressure it comes packaged in. A speaker's eagerness or anxiety is often felt by listeners as pressure to make them wrong or to change their way of thinking. As if it weren't hard enough to tone down one's own reactivity, doing so is often made even more difficult by the condition of the relationship.

How Some Speakers Make Us Hard of Hearing

We've all had experience with listeners whose emotional reactivity makes them defensive or argumentative instead of hearing what we're trying to say. An equally important barrier to understanding is the speaker's emotionality. A speaker who talks in a highly emotional way makes listeners anxious and therefore hard of hearing.

● ● ●

Some people have no idea how pressured and provoking their tone of voice is; they come at you like a bad dentist.

● ● ●

The hardest people to listen to are those who treat us with dictatorial disregard of our feelings. The pressured speaker may not know how he comes across, but his urgent, anxious tone of voice, emphatic hand gestures, or conclusion of every other statement with "Right?" (implicitly demanding agreement) makes us feel backed into a corner.

A Charged Atmosphere

The emotional climate between speaker and listener has a lot to do with the quality of understanding that can pass between them. If the atmosphere is calm, especially if it has a history of being calm, the listener can usually hear what the speaker is trying to get across. But if there's anxiety in the air—or even just intense feeling—the listener may be too tense to take in what's said. The listener may be anxious about being blamed, or pressured to change, or proven wrong. Speakers who trigger such feelings, venting emotion in a way that makes listeners feel backed against the wall, may not get heard, even though they have something important to say. It's the way hard things get said that determines whether or not they get heard.

The emotional state of a relationship depends not only on the way individuals express themselves but also on the extent to which they remain differentiated as individuals.

A differentiated individual is a mature and autonomous person who knows where his or her skin ends and other people's begin. In emotionally undifferentiated relationships anxiety becomes infectious and the partners increasingly reactive to each other, especially on hot subjects. Among some couples money is such a charged issue that sparks fly at the first mention of it. A mother who is poorly differentiated from her child may be so threatened by the childish retort "I don't love you!" that she either rescinds her rules or gets into a pointless discussion that begins with "But I love you." A more well-differentiated parent doesn't feel so threatened by her son's or daughter's protests. Such a parent has enough distance to realize that "I don't love you!" means "I'm angry that you won't let me have my way." Differentiation is achieved by learning to separate what you think from what you feel—and by learning to be yourself while respecting other people's right to be themselves.

When boundaries are blurred, individuals become emotionally fused and almost any agitation from the speaker will make a listener reactive. As differentiation decreases, individuality is less well defined, and emotional reactivity becomes more intense. Poorly differentiated and highly reactive people tend to come across as either emotionally demanding or avoidant.

An "independent" husband may be aware of his "dependent" wife's emotional reactivity but blind to his own. He sees her dependence because she shows it directly. When she objects to his wanting to go off by himself, he says, "You're so dependent! Why don't you develop some interests of your own and quit hanging on me?" She cries and accuses him of being selfish. As far as he's concerned, she's emotionally immature. She's so dependent that he can't even complain without her getting hysterical. What he doesn't see is how dependent *he* is on her feeling positively toward him, so much so that he's unable to hear her complaints as an expression of her feelings. He hears what she says only as a threat to himself and a constraint on what he wants to do. And so he goes off and broods in self-righteous resentment about his wife's inability to respond to him without reacting emotionally.

Gail had to talk to Leon about needing help around the house. She knew it was a sore subject because they'd both grown up with the expectation that housework was something wives did. But, damn it, with both of them working and the kids to look after, their family couldn't afford the luxury of a wife. For three months since starting her new job, Gail had put off asking Leon for help because she didn't want to start a fight. But she was finding it impossible to get dinner on the table before the kids started getting cranky, and so she just had to talk to him.

So that night after dinner Gail told Leon how unfair it was for her to have to do all the cooking and cleaning now that she was working. As she spoke, the anger and frustration she'd been sitting on for three months came pouring out.

Leon, who knew he wasn't doing his share, listened as Gail talked about how hurt she was that he hadn't offered to help. But as she went on about all she had to do and how little he did, Gail started talking faster and more pressured, waving her arms as though her words couldn't keep pace with her feelings. Leon listened with growing upset.

What started out as a legitimate request turned into a tirade. Instead of listening and feeling like cooperating, Leon felt attacked and got defensive. "Why do you have to go on and on about everything? And why do you have to exaggerate so: You do *everything*, and I do *nothing*. Who earns the real money in this family?"

That did it. Gail burst into tears, and Leon, who couldn't take it anymore, stormed out of the room and slammed the door. Gail was left alone crying in the living room, feeling how unfair it was that Leon was too selfish to care about her.

Sometimes a speaker's emotion generates anxiety in the listener, making it particularly difficult for the listener to be the receptive vehicle that the speaker requires. When it comes to telling your side, particularly in a relationship with a history of tension, the best way to be heard is to tone down your emotionality. Even if you don't make the mistake of blaming the other person, he or she may feel attacked if you express yourself in an anxious or pressured manner. The trouble is, sometimes it's hard not to.

• • •

We don't recognize the impact of our tone of voice, because we hear what we feel like, not what we sound like.

• • •

Elise gets annoyed because Jay takes the other side of almost every issue she brings up. This is a common complaint. Most subjects are complex enough to have two sides; when someone points to one side, we have a natural tendency to think of the other. The trouble is, it doesn't feel good to say the cup is half empty only to be told "No, it's half full." Jay's tendency to take the opposite position made Elise feel not just disagreed with but negated.

Once she commented that the neighbor's porch railing looked to be in bad shape and might break; someone might get hurt. Jay looked at the railing—which was in halfway good shape—and said, "I don't think so; it looks okay to me." When Elise said, "I hate it when you disagree with everything I say," Jay felt attacked. "Must I agree with everything you say?" he demanded. Like many reasonable married people, they discussed the issue without raising their voices or hearing each other.

Elise could understand Jay's feeling that it wasn't fair to have to agree with everything she said, but that wasn't what she wanted. She just wanted her feelings to be acknowledged. He heard that, sort of, but didn't know what he was supposed to do. "If you say the railing looks like it's going to break, and I don't think it is, how am I supposed to know that you're just expressing your feelings and that I'm only supposed to acknowledge them? How do I know what you want if you don't tell me?"

One reason Jay had trouble hearing Elise was that she expressed herself with anxious emotion. Even clear, meaningful messages were so charged with feeling that Jay reacted to her anxiety rather than to her statement. Instead of getting through to him, she became something to brace against.

Elise gets excitable and raises her voice because she's been holding things in and is eager to get them out. But when she gets anxious, Jay gets tense, and he's more aware of the knot in his stomach than of what Elise is trying to tell him. When she told him how much it bothered her that he always disagreed with her, it was the upset she conveyed that made him defensive, not the message.

No matter how they tried, Elise and Jay were never able to hear each other in heated discussions. Only when I interrupted and talked to them one at a time were they able to listen without a defensive response. It turned out that Elise had grown up with a father who demanded adherence to his rules and dismissed his children's opinions. Both Jay and Elise recalled her brother and his habit of responding to even the most insignificant disagreement as though it were a declaration of war: "Either you're with me, or you're against me!"

Jay and Elise aren't very different from many couples who sometimes despair of ever really being listened to by each other. If you want to be heard, consider how much emotionality and anxiety you have—or how much gets churned up when you talk about certain things. Listeners react to that emotion. If you can reduce your emotional pressure, you may get heard, even when the subject is difficult. Remember: it isn't so much what you say as how you say it that determines whether or not you get heard. That's one reason people are often more open to what they read than to what someone says to them. (At least I hope so.)

Let's take another look at the interaction between Jay and Elise. Jay had trouble hearing his wife because she expressed herself with anxious emotion, her sentences flapping at him like flags in a high wind. When her voice rankled and he shrank into himself, he didn't hear the sweet, eager girl he fell in love with but an echo of harshness from long ago. The "he" who was doing the hearing wasn't the part of him who was strong and loved his wife but a little boy part, the one who could never stand to hear that harsh and powerful voice telling him that he couldn't go out to play, that he had to stay in the house all afternoon buried alive in chores.

Is it men Medusa turns to stone, or the little boys inside them?

Hurt Feelings and Broken Connections

As a family therapist, I'm often consulted about impasses in relationships. Wives complain that their husbands don't care how they feel; husbands grumble that their wives nag; parents protest that their children avoid them; siblings insist that they're singled out unfairly; and adult children lament that they can't get close to their parents. Many of these individuals come to therapy by themselves because the people they're concerned about refuse even to talk about the problem.

Michael's sister Susan moved to the West Coast after a bitter divorce. When she called from Los Angeles to talk to him, her ex-husband, who just happened to have stopped by, answered the phone. Susan was furious. She felt betrayed and stopped speaking to her brother. When Susan didn't return Michael's phone calls, he got so upset that he took a plane to California the next day to straighten things out. But when he got there, Susan left town for the weekend because she wasn't ready to talk to him. Michael was livid. He could understand that she was upset, but he hadn't done anything wrong. And to refuse to see him after he had gone all the way to California—that he could not forgive.

The first step to healing a ruptured relationship is to understand the other person's point of view. Try to figure out what that person might be feeling and then say it in a way that invites him to elaborate. Until you acknowledge the other person's position, he is unlikely to be open to yours. He may listen, but he won't hear.

• • •

When you demonstrate a willingness to listen with a minimum of defensiveness, criticism, or impatience, you are giving the gift of understanding—and earning the right to have it reciprocated.

• • •

Michael tried to apologize to his sister, but his heart wasn't in it. After all, he hadn't done anything wrong. So although he said he was sorry she was upset, he just had to add that he hadn't done anything wrong. Unfortunately, when someone feels aggrieved, any attempt to justify your own behavior, no matter how innocent or well meaning, may cancel your acknowledgment of her feelings. Michael was infuriated when his sister refused to see him, but she rightly intuited that his attempt to make up carried the pressure for her to forgive him. If Susan had been less upset, Michael's attempts to heal the breach might have worked. But when some-one is really hurt, the only thing he or she wants to hear is an apology, not an apology loaded with self-justification. The greatest lesson in humility may be learning to say "I'm sorry I hurt you" without having to protest your innocence.

I saw Michael a total of three times over several months. In our first meeting I made exactly the same mistake I am preaching against here. Instead of acknowledging his resentment, I advised him to reach out to his sister. Since he felt that he'd already done so and been spurned, he rejected my advice.

Our second meeting occurred five months later. He'd been getting on with his life and had calmed down about the falling-out with his sister. Time and distance had softened his bitterness, and he was ready for suggestions about how to patch up the break. I advised him to write a letter acknowledg-ing the hurt and betrayal Susan felt and say that he was sorry. I cautioned him that the letter must be absolutely devoid of two elements that would render it ineffective: any hint of self-justification, expressed or implied, and any suggestion, expressed or implied, that his sister needed to do something about his apology. It had to be an unconditional apology—"I'm sorry I hurt you"—nothing more and nothing less. I also warned him that his sister's first response might be an angry one—something that can be hard to take when you apologize. He understood that and said he could accept it.

Four days after Michael wrote to his sister, he received a letter from her saying how betrayed she felt when her ex-husband answered the phone at her own brother's house. How could Michael have been so insensitive? After that Susan's letter lightened. She wrote about her job in California and a new friendship and asked Michael what he was up to. They've been on good terms ever since.

"He Never Talks to Me"

How can you be a good listener when certain people seem to withhold themselves from you and resist all your efforts at intimacy?

People are reticent in relationships because they don't want to get hurt. The introvert moves through life in a protective bubble of psychological distance not because his need for attention has ceased but because he's ceased to allow himself to feel it. Inside the prison of his defenses he preoccupies himself with other things. He keeps busy, he reads, he thinks, and he has long conversations in his head, where no one else can mess them up. Like many prisoners, he can be comfortable in his limited and protected routines, but the idea of parole into the wide world of other people and emotions terrifies him.

Although the emotional reticence of someone you care about can be powerfully frustrating, the reticent don't feel powerful. They feel vulnerable. People who withhold themselves from us are trying to insulate themselves from their own sensitivity to criticism or rejection. It isn't all them, either. In the process of trying to get closer to someone who doesn't say much, we often set up a pursuer–distancer dynamic.

Pursuers and Distancers

One of the most easily observed conversational patterns between intimate partners is the pursuer–distancer dynamic.[1]

As you may have noticed, pursuing distancers only makes them feel pressured and inclined to pull farther away. It's a dance between one person who moves forward and another who moves back. The pursuer–distancer dynamic is propelled by emotional reactivity—in both participants. The people who pull away from us aren't just "shy" or "withholding"; they're responding to the pressure with which we approach them. I can almost hear the protests: "I don't put any pressure on so-and-so; he [or she] just won't open up."

We rarely feel the emotional demands we put on others. What we feel is their response to it. The people who resist conversation with us may indeed be more reticent than most. Still, their backing off is not just habit but response.

Unfortunately, some of the people we find hardest to listen to are an important part of our lives: They are our partners, our parents, our chil-

---

[1]Thomas Fogarty, "The Distancer and the Pursuer," *The Family*, 1979, 7, 11–16.

dren, our bosses, or our colleagues, and they arouse our reactivity because our need endows them with the power to please and distress us. When the frustrations of trying to listen and be heard get to be too much, we may be tempted to give up.

Facing encounters that raise your anxiety tests your maturity, strengthens you if you have the courage to stand fast and let matters unfold, or weakens you if you fall back into reactivity and defensiveness. Making contact, letting others be themselves while you continue to be yourself, and learning to resist automatic reactions strengthens you and transforms your relationships. Staying open and staying calm—that's the hardest part. You do the best you can.

If all of this seems obvious—to listen well, you have to resist the urge to overreact—it's only obvious from an objective distance. Up close, when you're caught up in the pressure to get the words out or the aggravation of listening to someone saying something you don't want to hear, objectivity is in short supply. Emotionality takes over.

Exercises

1. Practice responsive listening twice in the coming week. First with someone who's easy to talk with. You probably won't be defusing an argument; you'll just be using responsive listening to draw the other person out a little more than usual. Second, pick someone you're likely to have a disagreement with. Plan in advance to use responsive listening and avoid giving your side of the argument until at least a day later.

2. To test your flexibility in a pursuer–distancer relationship, try the following for a week. If you are a pursuer, try backing off, and see what happens. Don't pout or get passive aggressive; just spend more time on your own. If you are a distancer, try initiating some mutually enjoyable activity before the pursuer has a chance to approach you.

   N.B. These experiments are not designed to cause any kind of permanent change in the pattern; they are merely experiments to help you explore the possibility of becoming more flexible.

3. To practice dealing with criticism, find an occasion to invite it. Plan in advance to respond without getting defensive. Listen without arguing. Invite the critic to say more. Then acknowledge what you think you heard and invite him or her to elaborate or correct your understanding.

Part Three

...

Getting Through
to Each Other

7

...

"Take Your Time— I'm Listening"

How to Let Go of Your Own Needs and Listen

Real listening requires *attention*, *appreciation*, and *affirmation*. You begin the process by tuning in to the other person, paying attention to what he or she has to say. Put no barriers between you. Turn off the TV, put down the newspaper, ask the kids to play in the other room, shut the door to your office. Look directly at the speaker and concentrate on what he or she is trying to communicate.

Practice listening whenever your partner, family member, friend, or colleague speaks to you, with the sole intention of understanding what he or she is trying to express. People need to talk—and be heard—to feel understood by and connected to you.

Paying Attention

You take the first step to better listening by making a conscientious effort to set aside whatever is on your mind long enough to concentrate on hearing what the other person has to say.

139

Listening to each other never seemed to be much of a problem for Tony and Joan before the baby was born. They had lots to talk about and, maybe more important, plenty of time for it. Then the baby came, and the pressures of parenthood squeezed the intimacy out of their relationship. They got out of the habit of going out together, and neither of them had much energy for conversation in their brief and hectic evenings at home.

Tony made an effort to ask Joan about her day, but when she responded only perfunctorily, he didn't pursue it. Anyway, he was so tired when he came home that he didn't really mind getting off by himself with the news-paper. They weren't angry or upset with each other, but they were drifting apart.

When Tony sought my advice about the lack of intimacy in the mar-riage, he described his failed attempts to talk to Joan at the end of the day. I could see two mistakes he was making. The first was timing. Trying to have a serious conversation when he first came in the door, while Joan was cooking supper and the baby was winding down like a little clock, just didn't work. The second thing was that Joan didn't respond well to global questions like "How was your day?" Such questions may work when someone is relaxed and ready to talk, but they aren't effective when some-one is worn out or distracted. Joan needed him to ask more specific ques-tions, like "How did it go at the pediatrician's?" or "What did the baby do today?"—questions specific enough to show that he was aware of what was going on in her life.

I did not, however, say any of this to Tony. Instead I turned to Joan and asked if she felt lonely. She said yes. Then I asked if she thought Tony was really interested in hearing what was going on with her. "Maybe ... ," she said softly, "but I don't feel it."

All I said to Tony was "I guess you better try harder."

• • •

Better listening doesn't start with a set of techniques. It starts with making a sincere effort to pay attention to what's going on in the other person's private world of experience.

• • •

My challenge to Tony—"I guess you better try harder"—turned out to be a one-session cure. He did try harder. It didn't occur to him to ask more specific questions; he just didn't give up so easily. Instead of offering Joan a brief moment's attention, he started showing real interest in her feelings and concern for her well-being. In response, she began to feel once again loved and cared for—and much more like being intimate with Tony in return.

When you're trying to have a conversation with someone who isn't revealing much of their thoughts and feelings, it may help to make empathic guesses about what's going on inside them. Comments like "Tough day?" or "Are you worried about something?" or "Is something bothering you?" may show enough awareness to make the other person feel that you're really interested. But it isn't any particular comment or technique that gets people to open up. It's taking a sincere interest in what they have to say. Listeners who pretend interest don't fool you for long—even though they sometimes fool themselves. The automatic smile, the hit-and-run question, the restless look in their eyes when you start to talk—all these are giveaways to the fact that they're more interested in being taken for good listeners than in really hearing what you have to say. Real listening means setting all that aside. Good listeners don't act needy. They don't charm, flatter, provoke, or interrupt. None of that *look at me, listen to me, admire me, appreciate me.* None of that. They suspend the self and listen.

Appreciating the Other Person's Point of View

Understanding one another is a give-and-take process. The best way to get the listening you need is to make the other person feel listened to first.

• • •

Most people aren't really interested in your point of view until they become convinced that you've heard and appreciated theirs.

• • •

Even when you're the one initiating a discussion, the best way to ensure that you'll be heard is to invite the other person to explain his viewpoint before you present yours. Suspending your agenda so as to hear the other person out enables you to understand what he thinks, helps make him feel understood, and clears the way for him to be more willing to listen to you.

Let the other person know you're interested in what he has to say by inviting him to say what's on his mind, what his opinion is, or how he feels about the issue under consideration—and then giving him your full attention.

"Can we talk about ... ? What do you think we should do?"

"I'm not sure I really understand how you feel about ... What is your point of view?"

"I'm sorry we had this misunderstanding. I'd really like to hear what happened as far as you're concerned."

"You seem upset with me. Am I right about that?"

Elicit the other person's thoughts and feelings about the subject at hand by asking specific questions that show your grasp of what she's said and encouraging her to elaborate.

"So what you're saying is ... Is that right?"

"I think I understand, but I want to make sure. You think we should ... ?"

"I'm not sure I know exactly what you mean. You said ... but I wish you'd say a little more about it so I'm sure I get it straight."

"I think I understand where we disagree, but I'm not sure. Did you mean that ... ?"

If you feel yourself getting impatient or defensive while the other person is talking, it's important to restrain your urge to respond until you've heard her out. Just keeping your mouth shut and pretending to listen may be better than interrupting, but it isn't the same as really listening. To really listen, try hard to appreciate what the other person is feeling. Imagine how you would feel if you were in her shoes.

• • •

When you're listening to someone but thinking about your own reactions, you're really talking to yourself, not listening.

• • •

Suspending your needs long enough to hear the other person out is part of being a good listener. But suspending your needs isn't the same thing as becoming a nonself.

Sometimes you need to recognize that you can't suspend your needs effectively unless you also find a way to fulfill them. So while it might seem selfish, telling your partner that you want to hear about his day but you have to get your own problem off your chest first may not be. By the same token, there are times when the most considerate and honest thing you can say to someone who wants to talk when you aren't up to listening is "I can't concentrate on what you're saying right now. Can we talk after supper?" Trying to listen when you're not up to it dries up your capacity to empathize.

Some listeners are so fearful of exerting their own individuality that they become nonselves, tucked into others, embedded in a framework of obligations and duties. These people find it easier to accommodate than to deal with conflict, threats of rejection, arguments, or signs of distress in others. Their anxious, demanding partners are frequently unaware of how much their mates accommodate to preserve harmony. They take it for granted and want more. Such compliant people may seem like good listeners, but you aren't really listening if you're nothing but a passive receptacle, a reluctant sponge.

● ● ●

Listening well is often silent but never passive.

● ● ●

Instead of listening passively, and maybe feeling a little trapped, get involved by asking questions that help the other person express his feelings or elaborate on what he's thinking.

"What does he do that bothers you the most?"

"What do you think she should do?"

"That sounds great! What was the best part?"

"What did you feel like saying to her?"

"What would you *have liked* to hear him say?"

Real listening means imagining yourself into the other's experience: concentrating, asking questions. Understanding is furthered not by knowing ("I understand") but by investigating—asking for elaboration, inquiring into the concrete particularity of the speaker's experience. The good listener isn't a passive receptor but an active, open one, attuned and inquiring.

When you ask the same old questions time after time—"What's new?" "How are you?"—you'll get the same old perfunctory answers. Here are some questions that suggest you're really interested in what's going on with someone.

"What's going on at work? At school? What are you working on?"

"What are you looking forward to this week? This month?"

"What are you worried about?"

"Tell me about your family."

"What's the thing that you're most enthusiastic about these days?"

"What do you love to do, and what are you good at doing?"

"What are you facing at home and at work?"

"What's been the highlight of your week so far?"

"What is it that you want to contribute? What is your value added? What do you bring to this situation?"

"Who are the people who influenced you most and how?"

"What dreams and ideas do you have? Are there any you've given up on?"

"What do you remember?"

"Tell me about some project that you're concerned about."

Affirming Your Understanding

Sometimes we pretend we're listening when we're not. In spite of this, we're taken aback when someone accuses us of not listening. One reason people wonder if we're listening is that we fail to let them know we heard them. Silence is ambiguous.

Without some sign of understanding, the speaker begins to wonder if what she's saying makes sense, if it's worth talking about. Doubts surface. *Maybe I'm boring him. Maybe I shouldn't be complaining like this.* Without some evidence of empathy, people don't trust us enough to tell us the simple truth about their feelings, much less reveal potentially dangerous truths. Everyone is vulnerable in this sense, and everyone holds back in some ways.

Ordinarily we take turns talking. The roles of speaker and listener alternate so naturally that it may seem artificial to call what one person says "the listener's response." Responding turns listeners into speakers. But listening well is a two-step process: First we take in what the speaker says, then we let him or her know it. Failure to respond is like an unanswered letter; you never know if you got through.

Repeating the other person's position in your own words is the best way to show that you understand. But effective listening is achieved not by summing up what the other person said as though that should be the end of it but as a means of inviting him to elaborate so that you can *really* understand.

• • •

Effective communication isn't achieved just by taking turns talking; it requires a concerted effort at mutual understanding.

• • •

The best way to promote understanding is to restate the other person's position in your own words, then ask her to correct or affirm your understanding of her thoughts and feelings. Remember: it isn't your paraphrase that's important; it's inviting the other person to expand on what he or she is saying. If you work on this process of feedback and confirmation until the other person has no doubt that you grasp her position, she will feel understood—and will then be more open to hearing from you.

"So you're saying you don't think Kevin should join Little League because it will put extra pressure on him and because you'll be the one who gets stuck driving him to all the games?"

"Let me make sure I understand what you're saying. You feel like you're always the one who calls to get together, and that makes you wonder if I really want to spend time with you. Is that right?"

"Okay, I want to make sure I understand. You're saying we should hire Gloria, but we should make it clear what we expect, and we should be serious about the probationary period, and if she doesn't do the job we should let her go at the end of six months. Have I got that right?"

"So all this time you've been thinking that I'm mad at you, and that's why you thought I didn't want to be affectionate. No wonder you're upset. You must have been feeling hurt for a long time."

"You Just Don't Get It, Do You?"

When one person says, "The world is round," and the other replies, "No, it's flat," it's clear that the second person got the first person's point and disagreed. But when the subject is more personal, disagreement—without some acknowledgment of the other person's point of view—can come across as invalidating the speaker's feelings. If people spoke in therapeutic jargon, they might say "I see what you're saying, but I don't agree." But since most of us not only don't speak like self-help manuals but often react in heat and haste, many conversations take on the form of two-part disharmony.

• • •

The simple failure to acknowledge what the other person says explains much of the friction in our lives.

• • •

The more heated the exchange, the more important it is to acknowledge what the other person says. When two people are talking about something important to them, each feels an urgent need to get his or her point of view across. Without some acknowledgment, each may continue to restate his or her position, thinking *If only he [or she] would listen to what I'm saying, we wouldn't have to keep arguing like this*.

One Friday night, after a long and tedious week, Sheila said, "We never go out." "That's not true!" said Rob, feeling attacked. "We went out last week." This just upset Sheila more, and she renewed her attempt to get Rob to understand what she was feeling. "You mean when we went with Linda and John for pizza? I don't call that going out. You never want to do anything but sit around in front of that stupid TV." Now Rob was pissed.

"I work hard all week, and if I want to relax on the couch, what's so wrong with that?" By this point Sheila felt completely invalidated. "You just don't get it, do you?" Then she went upstairs and slammed the bedroom door.

Maybe you can identify with Sheila. Or Rob. Or both of them. The choice between going out and vegging out is one that most of us have feelings about. But what was unfortunate in this quarrel that left both Sheila and Rob feeling so misunderstood was that neither took the time to acknowledge the other's point of view.

• • •

You don't have to be responsible for someone's feelings to acknowledge them.

• • •

When Sheila said, "We never go out," she was expressing a feeling—she's bored and lonely—and making a request: she wishes that she and Rob could have a little more fun, do something together, maybe be a little closer. But something about the way she said it (or he heard it) made Rob defensive. Instead of showing that he understood what she was feeling, he just felt criticized. He heard her saying that he was lazy, selfish, uninvolved—just the things he worries he might be—and so he didn't listen to her feelings, much less respond calmly to her request.

Dueling Points of View

When two people keep restating their own positions without acknowledging what the other one is trying to say, the result is dueling points of view. One is tempted—especially if one is a therapist—to think of two people involved in dueling declarations as simply lacking a communication skill, that of paraphrasing what your conversation partner says before responding. The trouble with this communication-as-skill perspective is that it leaves out conflict and anxiety, precisely the things that make understanding one another so difficult. The partners who don't acknowledge what each other says are afraid to. They're afraid that acknowledging the other's position means surrendering—"You're right and I'm wrong." Unfortunately, as in many vicious circles, their efforts to break through to each other by restating their own positions just locks misunderstanding in place.

When the subject isn't too emotional, the result is a mildly unsatisfying sense of at least having said what you mean, even if the other person didn't acknowledge it. But when feeling runs high, dueling declarations escalate into painful misunderstandings.

Professional advice givers often talk as though couples could get along fine if only they'd learn "to communicate"—making "I-statements" and all the rest. That's nice, but it overlooks the existence of real conflict.

Although they hadn't really discussed it, Charlotte assumed that when Hugh finished his PhD they would move back to New York. But Hugh liked where they were living, and when he announced that he might take a teaching job at the university, Charlotte felt betrayed.

Because the question of where to live was so important to both of them, they found it difficult to discuss without disparaging each other's point of view. When Hugh presented his arguments for staying, Charlotte would try to discredit them or say that he had a responsibility to make up to her the sacrifice she had made in leaving the city for the sake of his career. He'd respond by talking about the sacrifices he'd made for her. Later, after months of estrangement, Charlotte said that if at any point in the process Hugh had acknowledged that she had given up a lot for his schooling or had said that she would get her turn later, she could have agreed to stay. But instead of listening and acknowledging her right to feel the way she did, Hugh responded by saying that his career was more important than hers.

In another couple who faced the same issue, both wanted to move; the problem was where. Raymond was an accountant and Joyce was the dean of women at a small college. Both agreed that since he would be able to find work more easily, her search for another deanship should be given priority. Raymond, however, felt strongly about *where* he wanted to live. It wasn't so much a regional preference as wanting to live either in a big city or well out in the country—anything but suburbia, where Lawn Doctor reigned. And so half the time when Joyce told him that she'd read about a job opening, he'd respond by saying "I'd never live *there*." She'd feel defeated and angry and think he was being totally unreasonable.

Why did Hugh find it necessary to put Charlotte down by saying that his career was more important than hers? And why did Raymond have to reject so many of Joyce's possibilities so quickly? What made it so hard for these two husbands to acknowledge what their wives were feeling?

Hugh was apparently afraid that acknowledging Charlotte's feelings would automatically lead to giving in and acting on their dictates. Likewise, Raymond didn't seem to have the confidence that he could still say no to a potential new place after he and Joyce had visited it. Otherwise, why wouldn't he agree to at least take a look? Why weren't these two men able to listen better to their wives? Is it simply "selfishness" or "masculine insensitivity" or "immaturity" that prevents people from hearing each other? Maybe Hugh and Raymond had trouble listening to their partners because they felt anxious and insecure about their own ability to assert themselves. Maybe we—men and women—always have reasons for not listening, not understanding one another.

● ● ●

Listening is hard because it involves a loss of control— and if you're afraid of what you might hear, it feels unsafe to relinquish control.

● ● ●

He Says, She Says

He says, "You should have said something," she says, "You should have asked," and neither feels heard. She talks about the things she'd like to do, and he talks about being tired. He never hears what doing these things means to her, and she never hears that he hates his job. Arguments escalate, feelings go unrecognized, and minds don't meet as long as we fail to acknowledge what the other person says before we respond with what we have to say.

● ● ●

He says, she says—but neither acknowledges what the other says.

● ● ●

Behavior therapists teach couples to paraphrase what their partners say before going on to give their side. This is a device to interrupt the cross-complaining that keeps couples in conflict from ever feeling understood, much less actually doing anything about each other's complaints. If a husband tells his wife that he wishes she would cook something different for supper, and she complains that he's impossible to please—and he gets defensive and withdraws to brood over how unfair she is—neither one of them will feel understood. This misunderstanding—and many others like it—has less to do with being unable to resolve conflict than with being unable to tolerate it. If instead of getting defensive and attacking, either person would simply acknowledge what the other said, it might not prove so difficult to come together.

Even when conflict is serious, we all feel better if we can at least say how we feel—what bothers us, what we wish—and have the other person say those magic words: "I understand."

Many of the people I talk to have less than ideal sex lives. Maybe mine is a biased sample, but most of the people I see who've been married for ten years or more have sex maybe once a month, maybe less. Even in therapy, few people mention this issue. Not only are they embarrassed (most people assume that most other people are successful parents and have happy sex lives), but also they've given up hope. Why talk about something so personal and painful when all their previous efforts have only made them angry and ashamed?

Once they find the courage to talk about problems in their sexual relationship, some couples are able to make changes for the better, while others aren't. But almost all feel better for talking about it. What makes them feel better, even if nothing changes, is being able to say how they feel, what they don't like, what they wish, and to admit feeling inadequate—something each partner inevitably feels and generally doesn't realize the other one feels.

Why do people need a therapist to have these conversations? They don't. *If* they can each say how they feel about the situation, and the other can hear *and acknowledge* these feelings before going on to say how he or she feels.

Most of us are reactive when it comes to sex, but some people are reactive to so many things that they fail to acknowledge what anyone says about anything. If you complain to such people that they always argue with everything you say, they may protest that you're asking them to always agree with you. They're not aware that it takes some kind of acknowledgment of what you're saying for you to feel not agreed with but heard.

The Importance of Relinquishing Control

As I've said, I don't like to be interrupted in the middle of a story by someone giving advice I didn't ask for or "sharing" a similar experience. Interruption is interruption. What's missing is some expression of understanding, something like "Gee, that's lousy." What's going on in both cases—and others—is that the listener won't relinquish control of the exchange. Many of us are convinced that we're good listeners because we say all the right things. But are we? Often the speaker ends up feeling unheard, because what we're really doing is going through the motions.

"Why Don't You Just ... ?"

A wise supervisor once told me that my treatment of a shy, overweight young man was bogged down because I was trying to change him before he felt understood by me. To me it seemed so simple: if the young man would only make a little effort to initiate conversations with people, at the same time we explored the roots of his insecurity, he could work toward change on two fronts. He, however, felt that my suggesting that he simply start doing what he found so difficult proved that I didn't understand how painfully self-conscious he was. The supervisor's technical recommendation (which had to do with transference and countertransference) was: "Shut up and listen."

A Gaping Silence

If everyone followed my supervisor's advice, the world would be a better place. But if listening were only a negative accomplishment, you could concentrate (as many therapists, and people playing therapist, do) on simply not interrupting. Speakers may be gratified at being allowed to say what's on their minds but frustrated by the absence of curiosity and appreciation. This means that, taken too literally, "shut up and listen" isn't enough to convey understanding. If you're telling someone at a party about what kind of work you do and she's listening without interrupting, but her eyes are wandering around the room, you hardly feel listened to.

Whether or not someone is really listening only that person knows. But, on the other hand, if you don't feel listened to, you don't feel listened to. We judge whether or not others are listening to us by the signals we see. Are they showing that they're paying attention by setting aside distractions and turning toward us?

Before they comment on what we're saying, people show interest and attention by maintaining eye contact, smiling with pleasure or frowning with concern, and making little interjections like "uh-huh" and "really?" Head nods also show attention; larger and repeated ones show agreement. You don't have to take Elementary Clinical Methods to learn these responses; they follow from taking an interest.

The Leading Question

Questions convey interest, but sometimes the interest they convey is tangential to what the person is trying to say. Sometimes the distraction is obvious. If you're telling a friend all the inconsiderate things your husband did on your vacation and she interrupts with a lot of questions about where you stayed, you won't feel listened to. At other times people seem to be following but can't help trying to steer. These listeners impose their own narrative structures on our experience. Their questions assume that our stories should fit their scripts: "Problems should be denied or made to go away"; "Everyone should be together"; "Men are insensitive"; "Bullies must be confronted." By finishing our sentences, pumping us with questions, and otherwise pushing us to say what they want to hear, controlling listeners violate our right to tell our own stories.

Guidelines for Good Listening

1. Concentrate on the person speaking.
   - Set aside distractions.
   - Suspend your agenda.
   - Interrupt as little as possible. If you do interrupt, it should be to encourage the speaker to say more.
2. Try to grasp what the speaker is trying to express.
   - Don't react to just the words—listen for the underlying ideas and feelings.
   - Try to put yourself in the other person's shoes.
   - Try to understand what the other person is getting at.

3. Let the speaker know that you understand.
   - Use silence, reassuring comments, paraphrasing.
   - Offer empathic comments.
   - Make opening-up statements (tell me more, what else) versus closing-off statements (I get it; the same thing happened to me).

How to Get the Listening You Deserve

(The devil just whispered in my ear that maybe I should make that "... the Listening You Want." Maybe we already get the listening we deserve. But I'm not going to listen to that old devil.)

How to Ask for Support Without Getting Unwanted Advice

One way to get the listening you need is to tell people what you want.

"I'm upset and I need to talk to you. Just listen, okay?"

"I have a problem I need to discuss, but I'm not ready to decide what to do, so it would be helpful if you could just listen to me."

If you don't want a reactive or intrusive response, anticipate your listener's expectations.

"I'm not asking you to agree with me, but can you understand where I'm coming from?"

"I want to tell you something and I don't want you to get mad at me. Just listen and think about what I'm saying, will you?"

"I want your opinion about something, but I'll have to figure out what I want to do about it. Will you give me some advice, even if I don't end up following it?"

If someone gives advice when you just want to be listened to, by all means say so. But put the emphasis on what you want, not on how intrusive she is: "Thanks for the advice, but right now I just want to tell you about what happened" works better than "I didn't ask for any advice," or "Can't you just listen for once, without always having to tell me what to do!"

How to Handle Interruptions

If you're driving down the road and someone cuts in front of you, there's not much you can do about it. Oh, you can hit your horn and call that person a certain member of the canine family if you wish. But you pretty much have to yield unless you want to get into an accident. The same isn't true when somebody cuts in when you're talking. You can't be interrupted unless you allow it. When you're talking, you have the right of way.

If someone starts to interrupt, you can:

- Hold up your index finger.

- Say "Wait a minute, I'm not finished."

- Just keep talking: "What I was trying to say is ... "

If someone does cut you off:

- Instead of getting upset (or instead *of just* getting upset), practice saying "I wasn't finished; please hear me out." Then go back to what you were saying and finish saying it.

- Comment on feeling cut off, but without lecturing or attacking:

    "I wish you'd let me finish what I was saying."

    "I'm sorry, but I can't pay attention to your story because I wasn't finished telling mine."

    "I was trying to tell you something that's important to me. When you start talking about something else out of the blue, I feel like you're not interested in me or what I have to say."

    "I was listening to that story on the news. I wish you'd wait a minute before breaking in."

How to Listen to People Who Aren't Easy to Listen To

If you're unlucky enough to know someone who's always talking about himself or herself, you might appreciate some advice about how to change that person. The best I can offer is the suggestion to think systemically.

People who talk too much are difficult to endure, but their need for our attention is genuine. Their neediness is a burden, but they shouldn't be made to feel ashamed of it. Shaming people for their needs makes them feel worse and intensifies the need. Even if you don't criticize someone for talking too much, not listening to them has an isolating effect, which only increases their need to be heard.

When we describe someone as self-centered or say that he's always talking about himself, we are in fact describing only half of a relationship. In forty years of counseling couples, I've met very few people who don't think they do an unequal share of listening in their relationships. This isn't to say that there aren't people who talk about themselves more than others, but if we turn away from the needs of those we love, we are part of the problem.

One of the secrets to dealing with the difficult people in your life is to figure out how to play the hand you're dealt, rather than fretting about what that hand is. The reason some people in our lives remain one-dimensional is that that's as far as we go with them. Part of the reason your father-in-law always wants to talk about himself is that you rarely listen, or you listen halfheartedly. As long as he feels unlistened to, he's unlikely to have much interest in what anyone else has to say. If instead of stewing in the trapped anxiety of someone with nothing to do but flinch, you listen a little more to someone who talks too much, you might find the balance of the relationship shifting. Even a small shift can make a big difference.

Resisting the Temptation to Turn Away

At times when we want to control others' access to us, we may avoid looking at them. A man watching television may avoid looking at his wife when she tries to speak to him. Similarly, a waitress may evade a customer's glance to prevent his initiating a request she's too busy to fulfill at the moment.

A paradoxical example of this responsive unavailability occurs in psychoanalysis, where the analyst sits behind the recumbent patient. The result is disconcerting. Unable to see how the therapist is responding, the patient is unsure of being understood and sympathized with. The therapist may feel equally uncomfortable in not being able to offer visible evidence of interest. Eventually, this constrained arrangement turns out to be liberating. The patient, who gets to trust that he won't be interrupted, learns to follow his own thoughts more fully and to express them more freely. The therapist discovers that looking away with no pressure to demonstrate interest enables him or her to listen more freely and to think about what's being said.

What is to be learned from the analyst being liberated to listen by not having to appear attentive? We've noted that listening well means suspending our needs, including the need to *do* something—to solve problems, to say the right thing, even to act attentive. Better to *be* attentive. Be interested. Listen hard. Overcome the need to get credit for listening.

It may not be possible in everyday life to offer that perfect and silent listening in which analytic patients are encouraged to reveal and reconstruct themselves. If people have learned not to expect careful listening from you, you may have to reassure them of your interest. But if you listen carefully, people will learn to trust you. Just listening, without interrupting or turning away, goes a long way toward establishing that trust.

Exercises

1. The next time someone you care about has something to say, give him or her your full attention for three minutes. How long did those three minutes seem? How hard was it to stay tuned? How hard did you have to work to suppress what you wanted to say? What were the consequences of devoting that time to listening?

2. Note the next time someone responds to you with advice instead of listening. Write down later how you felt and why you think he or she couldn't hear you out.

3. Is there someone you can listen to without jumping in with advice or correction? If so, why? Does it have anything to do with respect?

8

...

"I Never Knew You Felt That Way"

Empathy Begins with Openness

Among the unhelpful expectations we bring to listening are preconceived notions about what the speaker is going to say and how communication should take place. Assuming you know what someone is going to say means you don't have to bother to listen.

Our assumptions about how people should talk to each other aren't usually conscious; they're part of the way we were brought up. Assuming that your way of communicating is the right one means you'll have trouble relating to people with different conversational styles and sensitivities. Such assumptions come in pairs of opposites, such as:

"Polite people make requests indirectly" versus "Honest people say what they want."

"Explanations should be short and sweet (rambling on is boring)" versus "Explanations should be thorough and complete (make sure the other person understands what you mean)."

The listener who settles for confirming his expectations is like the museum-goer who looks at paintings only long enough to verify the name of the artist; he'll never get closer to another person's experience. There is no bridge of understanding, no touching. The listener who remains open, on the other hand, sometimes experiences surprise and delight as his assumptions topple and he discovers the speaker—child, lover, friend—in a deeper, fuller way.

● ● ●

The essence of good listening is empathy, achieved by being receptive to what other people are trying to say and how they express themselves. Empathy takes a mind open to other sensibilities.

● ● ●

Although most people would improve their listening by setting aside preconceived notions and remaining receptive to what others are trying to say, a complete absence of assumptions is neither possible nor desirable. Anticipation is useful. Anticipating how someone might react can help you express yourself more effectively; anticipating a speaker's needs and style of communicating can help you hear all levels of messages being sent. So, what am I saying? Are expectations a help or a hindrance to listening?

Expectations hinder communication when they take the form of fixed assumptions and egocentric perspectives. Such expectations are unexamined and close us to other points of view. Expectations promote communication when they take the form of sensitivity to other people's styles of communicating. Such sensitivities make us aware, thoughtful, and receptive, not biased.

Creating a Climate of Understanding

One of the most common expectations we bring to conversational encounters, especially at home, is that we will be able to communicate by doing what comes naturally. Unfortunately, the listening we do on automatic pilot is often perfunctory, precisely the kind of halfhearted listening that makes our relationships less fulfilling than they could be. If you want to make any relationship more rewarding, practice *responsive listening*.

Responsive listening means hearing the other person out, then letting him know what you understand him to be saying. If you're right, the speaker will feel a grateful sense of being understood. If you didn't quite get what he intended to say, your feedback allows him another chance to explain.

Responsive listening can be practiced like any other skill if you're willing to put in the effort. If.

Listening Takes Practice

Why is it that we can admit we don't dance well or can't draw, but we won't admit (even to ourselves) that we aren't good at listening? Because being a good listener doesn't seem like a skill; it seems like a character trait, related to being a nice person, someone interested in others. If you're not a good tennis player, it's because you haven't practiced. If you're not a good listener, you're a bad person.

Think of how many situations where familiarity, tension, or distraction has made you fail to be attentive, considerate—concerned. The next time your partner comes home at the end of the day, or your child runs to tell you something, or someone at work wants to talk, try making an extra effort to be attentive. Paying attention goes a long way. Your effort to listen a little longer and more carefully to others will initiate a positive spiral in all of your relationships.

"I Know What You're Going to Say"

"Like hell, you do!" Have you ever felt like saying that when someone finishes your sentence?

• • •

**The person who starts a sentence
should be the one to finish it.**

• • •

Unfortunately, jumping to conclusions is something we all do at times. You may not actually make the remark I've used as a head for this section, but one of the bad listening habits we all need to break is making assumptions about what people are going to say.

Rachel got home at six-thirty instead of six as she'd promised and said, "I'm sorry I was late, I—"

"That's okay," Patrick broke in to say, "the kids and I made spaghetti. It's all ready."

Rachel was grateful not to have to cook supper but still felt cut off. She was about to say that she was late because her boss dumped a last-minute assignment on her, but Patrick's assumption that she was about to apologize for inconveniencing him made her feel that he didn't care. All he was interested in, it seemed to her, was his supper.

She could have told him anyway, right? Maybe. But if he's in the habit of cutting her off, she may get tired of trying to force him to listen to her.

Cutting someone off to take over conversational control can certainly be annoying, but so can jumping in before a speaker is finished with words of encouragement or agreement or to tell a similar story.

At first Hank appreciated Sharon's habit of interjecting little expressions of support when he talked to her. Her *wows, gees,* and *what a shames* made him think she was tuned in to his feelings. But after a while these expressions seemed trite and predictable. They began to make him feel that she was more interested in coming across as supportive than in really listening to him.

Being supportive means neither anticipating nor exceeding a speaker's own expression of feeling. I knew a woman who was so supportive that waves of compassion radiated from her like hot air from an oven. She may have been trying to be sensitive, but after a while I was reminded of the Al Franken refrain: "You're good enough, you're smart enough, and doggone it, people like you!"

"Oh, I know what you mean!" Celia said. "My principal treats me the same way." Though she intended to establish empathy, Todd was annoyed. He doubted that her principal really gave her as many last-minute assignments as his boss gave him. Besides, that wasn't his point. He never got to make his point because Celia cut him off to demonstrate that she understood.

The best way to avoid cutting people off is to concentrate on what they're trying to say. Give them a chance to make their point, acknowledge it, and *then* say your piece. Don't pounce at the first pause. Curb the impulse to switch the focus to you and what's on your mind. Don't tell every story that crops into your head. (I wince as I write this.) Stop and consider whether your comment would encourage the speaker to say more or take over the conversation.

"When Is It My Turn?"

Sometimes we don't listen because we've developed habits that interfere with openness. We make assumptions, we react emotionally, and we focus on what we have to say. We seem to be listening, but we can't resist giving our feelings, our experience, our advice, our opinion.

How do you overcome focusing on what you have to say? Make an effort. Often what you have to say is fine, but it skips hearing and acknowledging what the other person was saying.

Not: "I hate my job."
"Yeah, me too."

But: "I hate my job."
"Gee, that's too bad. What's going on?"

Always listen first. Then acknowledge what the other person said. Whether and when you take a turn depends on whether the relationship is one of equals. If your child complains, usually just listen. If it's a friend, listen first, then tell your story. But "equals" aren't equal when one person is upset. That person gets preference. It's like when someone you live with gets sick. He or she needs the attention. Put your needs on hold.

Not: "I felt all alone when you left me at your office party for a half hour to talk to your boss."
"What could I do? He pays my salary. He wanted to talk. I had no choice."

But: "I felt all alone when you left me at your office party for a half hour to talk to your boss."
"I'm sorry."

If you make a habit of talking out of turn, people will consider you intrusive. If you get excited and jump in before the other person has finished, try to catch yourself and back off politely. Say "Go ahead" or "I'm sorry, I didn't let you finish."

Even if you *do* know what somebody is going to say, he or she still needs to say it—and have you acknowledge it—before feeling understood. If conversation were an aerial dogfight, it would be wise to anticipate the other person's moves so you could shoot them down as fast as possible. But conversation shouldn't be like that. The person who has something to say wants to express both an idea and a feeling. Listening with an open mind gives you a chance to discover what's on her mind and gives her a chance to clarify her own thinking and feeling. The gift of your attention allows you to understand—and the other person to *feel* understood.

How to Move Beyond Assumptions to Openness and Empathy

The psychoanalyst Wilfred Bion said that to listen well you must "set aside memory, desire, and judgment."[1] This is a formula for openness, calling as it does for listeners to suspend preconceptions, assumptions, and their own needs. Real listening is an act of self-transcendence.

However much the people in our lives care about us, they're still largely preoccupied with their own agendas: worries, problems, projects, grudges, hopes, dreams. Even (or especially) if unspoken, such personal agendas are compelling and absorbing. As long as they remain private, these preoccupations have a tendency to separate us from each other. Shared thoughts and feelings are a step toward each other. Empathy is the bridge.

An empathic listener inquires and acknowledges what we're thinking and feeling and thus confirms our experience. In this way the receptive listener vitalizes us by emotional participation and reflection—feeding back to us what we sometimes experience as inchoate.

People live in their own personal and subjective worlds. To meet, truly meet, means that they must open up parts of themselves and share them. And they must be received. Much of the time we hide away our real feelings, sometimes even from ourselves. As a result, our conversational

---

[1]Wilfred Bion, *Transformations* (New York: Jason Aronson, 1983).

encounters, like our relationships themselves, often consist of shadows dancing with each other.

Empathy bridges the gap between us, but it requires an effort at openness. Too many assumptions are inimical to understanding. You can hardly take in anything like the full richness of someone else's experience if you're just waiting for your turn. Empathy takes restraint; it takes work.

The empathic listener offers a bond of understanding in a deep sense. It's more than the dutiful sympathy you might get from your hairdresser. It's a deeper resonance of understanding. Perhaps you remember a time when you were hurt or scared and a friend put a hand on your shoulder. Empathy is like that.

Empathic listening means working a little harder at understanding the other person before asking him to do the same for you. It means demonstrating your understanding with comments that draw out the other person's thoughts and feelings: "Uh-huh," "I see," "Yes." Simple empathic comments express understanding and help bring out something unexpressed in the other person's experience. This helps break down the withholding of feeling that keeps us apart. Withholding is unnecessary with someone who cares and understands.

● ● ●

The empathic listener celebrates the naturalness of what is felt—"No wonder you were mad!"—and helps to overcome the other person's tendency to hold back.

● ● ●

Empathy is achieved by suspending your assumptions and placing yourself attentively at the service of the other person, being alert to what he or she is saying and to the emotional subtext. It means listening without being in a hurry to take over.

Empathy requires two kinds of activity. The first is receptive openness, like a moviegoer who allows himself to be absorbed in a film and moved by the actors. The second is a balance between thinking and feeling. This requires a deliberate shift from feeling *with* a speaker to thinking *about* her. What is she saying? Meaning? Feeling?

Suppose your mate comes home and says he's had a bad day. You know what that feels like. You're sympathetic. So you ask what happened. He says he has to go out of town next week. His boss wants him to represent the agency at a meeting in Buffalo, and he's not looking forward to it.

You know how he feels. All that travel. And Buffalo of all dreary places!

Maybe that's how *you'd* feel. You don't look forward to business trips because you don't like to be away from home.

Our own feelings make us sympathetic. But empathy, real empathy, requires a second step: thinking *about* the other person. How does his "not looking forward" feel?

Maybe he's excited about being chosen to speak for the agency. It's a chance to show the boss he can handle more responsibility. But maybe that makes him nervous. Speaking in public is a lot harder when your agenda is trying to prove yourself.

Whether or not your partner gets to talk about these issues, to clarify and share his feelings, depends on how empathically you listen. If you want to know how someone feels, ask, and then listen.

• • •

**Do you rely on sympathy and presume you understand,
or do you use empathy and work at it?**

• • •

Remaining open to what other people have to say is easier in the absence of conflict. Being at odds with someone means that you have your own agenda, and the conflict makes you anxious to press your point of view. But since two force fields can't occupy the same space at the same time, even if your only objective is to get your ideas across, the most effective way to do so is to hear the other person out first—make him feel understood and taken into account. Here are a couple of examples:

A few years ago a colleague who was editing a book on psychoanalytic therapy changed jobs and asked me to take over for him. I was delighted— until I saw that most of the chapters weren't very good. It was hard for me, a young and relatively unknown psychologist, to convince the authors, who were big shots, to do the necessary work. One of the authors, however, was very solicitous. He called every week to ask how the book was coming and even offered to be my coeditor. Then I read his chapter. It wasn't the worst, but it was close. Trying to be diplomatic, I returned the manuscript, praising its strong points and asking for a few minor changes. Three months went by. Then I received a letter thanking me for my "suggestions" but saying that a couple of his friends had read over his chapter and agreed with him that it was just fine the way it was. Arghh!

After counting to ten (about twenty times), I wrote saying that he seemed upset about something and I was interested in hearing about it. He called the day he received my letter and told me with a lot of feeling how hard he'd worked on his chapter and how much rewriting the previous editor had already put him through. I didn't really have to say anything. He was so appreciative of my listening to him that as soon as he finished complaining he thanked me for being understanding and said he'd be glad to make the changes I'd asked for.

Frankly, I hadn't really been interested in this man's feelings, but to be able to negotiate with him, I had to hear him out first, or he never would have been receptive.

With someone you do care about, empathic openness is more than a useful strategy. It's the essential means of discovering what things look like from inside that person's world.

Linda knew Andrew didn't like to spend time with her. He was married to his career. That's why she'd developed so many outside interests over the years. Now that the children had gone off into the wide world, Linda began to sense the marriage entering its second death. Maybe it was time to turn off the life supports. She dreamed of freedom. What had she expected when she married? Attention, shared interests, affection, conversation. What she had was what she did on her own.

And Andrew? After years of professional success, he was becoming a failure at loneliness. He longed to be closer to Linda, to share something more than domestic arrangements. He dreamed of love. Unfortunately, they'd gotten out of the habit of talking. He went about his business wearing the armor of indifference.

When Linda came to see me—maybe a therapist would tell her what she wanted to hear—I tried to point out one reason she felt stuck: she wasn't open to the possibility of trying to talk to her husband, trying to rekindle some basis for staying together other than sharing children.

Linda had assumed that nothing would change and so it would be a waste of time talking to Andrew. When Linda tried to open up and talk to Andrew, she found out that he had assumed she no longer wanted to be involved with him, so he didn't say anything.

Such assumptions are protective. They keep us from getting our hopes up and our feelings hurt. But they also keep us from getting through to each other.

• • •

Most of our assumptions about why communication breaks down are about the other guy. We take our own input for granted.

• • •

After their talk Linda and Andrew did get a little closer. Not a lot, but enough to make a difference. Shared understanding was the first step.

Openness may be the key to listening, but not total openness, as in a blank screen. Real receptivity must be informed by sensitivity to other people.

Sensitivity: Expectations at Their Best

One of the things we learn after a while—sometimes a long while—is that different people have different emotional needs. If, for example, you need time alone when you're upset, it might be hard to remember that in the same circumstances the first thing your partner wants is to talk. People also have different ways of communicating. To be a good listener you have to be sensitive to other people's conversational styles. The automatic rhythms and nuances of a person's conversational style include such things as whether descriptions are detailed or abbreviated, whether the pace of speaking is fast or slow, and whether who-said-what-to-whom or what-I'm-working-on-now is the preferred topic.

To Naomi, loud, overlapping talk was an indication of enthusiasm and mutual involvement. To Wardell, it was a sign of rudeness and not listening.

Hannah wants details; Ivan feels interrogated.

Rick wants Sherry to get to the point. To her it feels like he isn't interested in what she has to say.

Veronica likes to talk things over. She complains that Chet is always leaving the room. Chet replies that Veronica says something and he responds, then when he goes to finish what he was about to do, she gets mad.

Listening between intimates often erodes over time because the only way they know to solve problems is to talk things out. But when communication styles clash, talking doesn't help. Trying harder, if it means doing more of the same, only makes matters worse.

People who communicate indirectly feel that people close to them should understand how they feel. Direct communicators think, "We should be able to tell each other what we want."

Being sensitive to other people's conversational ways doesn't mean you have to have them all figured out. It means you should be receptive. If you're used to a New York City pace and you're listening to a languid southern speaker whose conversation is like an old hound dog that stops at every tree, relax. Be patient. You might even get to enjoy the differences.

Unfortunately, when conversational styles differ, misunderstandings multiply. It's difficult to straighten out such differences if you're convinced of the rightness of your position and the wrongness of the other's.

Belinda was with her husband at a New Year's Eve party at his parents' house. Halfway through the evening, Belinda's mother-in-law came over and whispered, "Loosen up, have some fun. Don't be so formal!"

Belinda was annoyed. She had been having fun. She'd had several enjoyable conversations with her husband's cousins. She wasn't being formal; she was being herself.

Belinda was pissed. *Who does that woman think she is? Did I say anything to her about cackling hysterically whenever anybody said something?* In fact, Belinda found the mother-in-law's loud show of emotion and high-pitched chatter jarring. It wasn't her style.

Both of these people were behaving in self-evidently appropriate ways, the ways they were brought up to behave.

Some people consider their restrained style of speaking "polite." They find people with a more expressive style "crude," "loud," "histrionic," "vulgar." More emotive speakers think of themselves as "open and honest," "warm," "friendly," while they think of more restrained speakers as "aloof," "standoffish," "distant."

(Notice, incidentally, how Belinda and her mother-in-law each addressed their differences in character. The mother-in-law was "honest" or "rude," depending on your point of view. Belinda was "polite" or "aloof," as you see it.)

Sensitivity means being responsive to other people's feelings. It doesn't mean assuming you know what they're going to say; it means being interested enough to find out. On the other hand, sensitivity does mean using your knowledge of other people to understand their perspective and respect their individuality.

Some of the ways you can show sensitivity are:

- Paying attention to what the other person is saying
- Acknowledging the other person's feelings
- Listening before giving an opinion
- Listening without offering advice
- Listening without immediately agreeing or disagreeing
- Noticing how the other person appears to be feeling—and then asking
- Asking about his or her day, both before and after
- Respecting a person's need for quiet times
- Respecting a person's need to address problems
- Listening to but not pushing too hard for feelings

• • •

Maybe you *won't* get through to some people as long as you keep approaching them the same way you always do.

• • •

We're Most Insensitive to Those We Love

What makes someone insensitive to what others are saying? To figure out why a listener becomes reactive instead of listening, consider where the person's anxiety might be coming from. Sometimes anxiety comes from stress—real or imagined. People resist both actual and threatened change. We think of powerful people as dominating relationships and perhaps therefore not willing to listen, but in fact it's often the powerless who have trouble listening. A man who feels that his opinions about the children aren't respected may resist his wife's efforts to talk about them. A woman who doesn't feel entitled to say what she wants (and doesn't want) may resist her husband's attempts to discuss sex. Most people begin to listen better once they realize what power they do have in a relationship.

On the other hand, sometimes a person who clearly seems to have power in a relationship—a parent, say, or a dominating spouse—still doesn't listen. When a dominant person doesn't listen, it's usually because some hidden emotional issue is present, making him or her anxious.

One afternoon Tommy came home from school with so much restless energy that he decided to mow the lawn. The machine plowed into the deep grass, releasing its familiar sweet smell. But Tommy hadn't gone ten feet when the mower stalled, its blade clogged with wet grass. After several frustrating starts and stops, he shoved the insubordinate machine back into the garage, stomped into the house cursing and banging, went upstairs, and slammed his door.

By this time Tommy's parents were home. When his father asked what was the matter, Tommy told him about his lousy day at school, then coming home and the lawn mower not working. He was frustrated and angry.

Instead of empathizing, his father gave him a lecture. "When you have a problem, it doesn't do anybody any good to lose control and start yelling. You have to stop and be calm. Nothing is accomplished when you get upset." As his father went on, Tommy's head sank slowly to his chest.

"You can't cut grass when it's a foot high and be in a hurry. You've got to go through it very, very slow. You can't bull your way through anything—including life."

Tommy tried to explain. "Yeah, but when you've had a bad day at school and you come home and everything goes wrong, your anger keeps building. You've got to let it out somehow."

"Remember what we talked about last night? About problems? What did I say?"

"You said you've got to swallow your tongue." Tommy had stopped looking for sympathy and was now just trying to hang on to some of his pride.

But his father wasn't finished. "I also told you that problems when they're compounded make bigger problems. But if you take that problem and break it down, and make individual problems out of it, you can usually solve them very easily. Remember we talked about that?"

Tommy gave up trying to explain himself, and the conversation was finished.

This is a story of a father's failure to listen. The father asks his son why he's upset and then, when the boy tries to tell him, instead of listening, gives him a speech on the futility of anger, a lecture for a course the boy didn't sign up for. Tommy attempted to explain his feelings because he was looking for understanding. Instead he became a captive audience forced to listen to an account of his own inadequacies.

What's so hurtful in this encounter (and others like it) isn't that the father has a different perspective from his son; it's that, because of the feelings his son's behavior arouses in him, he tries to allay his own anxieties by pushing his perspective on the boy. In this scenario, Father knows best; Tommy's perspective carries no weight. It's never even acknowledged. The real impact of Father's lessons for living may be that Tommy grows up to be one of those people, like his father, with didactic views on everything—and unable to listen.

But *why* was Tommy's father so unable to listen to him explain why he was upset? What was so threatening? Anger.

Emotional intolerance is a huge impediment to listening. Some people, like Tommy's father, are so reactive to anger that they can't tolerate even normal amounts of this basic human emotion. Other people are just the opposite: at the slightest provocation they flare up like a lit match. In the next chapter we'll see how to cope with anger and how to keep it from spoiling listening.

It's sad that we're so reactive to the people closest to us. The closer the relationship, the more engaged our own needs, and the more we need, the harder it is to be receptive.

Sensitivity to Other People's Inner Voices

One example of failing to be sensitive to other people's need to be heard is giving unwanted advice. When you're tempted to give advice, remember those conflicting inner voices. Doing so may not only stop you from wasting your breath (and credibility) but also might give you a fresh perspective on the person's feelings and how to approach him or her about a sensitive issue.

What if the issue has already touched off a tirade? The ideal response to the person who goes into a rage about something is to acknowledge what he's feeling. Something's bothering him, and he's trying to tell you that. But there are times when most of us find it impossible to listen to someone who's shrieking at us. And so the question becomes not how to defuse the blowup but how to repair things afterward. That's when thinking about the other person's rage and your reaction in terms of subpersonalities can help you gain a little empathy and insight. Seeing a person's tirade as a childish tantrum may help you figure out that he feels weak and helpless, not powerful. Powerful people don't scream. But if screaming scares you (welcome to the club), when you calm down, if you consider what kind of person the screaming reduced you to (a scared kid, say), that in itself may help you recover your objective adult self when it comes to addressing the incident later.

"Have You Got a Minute?"

One way to use sensitivity to *get* better listening is by checking to see if the person you want to talk to is busy. People signal their openness to conversation by their posture. The person who looks up expectantly when you enter the room or walks up to you and says hello is probably open to talking. The person with her head down, looking away when you approach, or reading, intent on the TV, or otherwise preoccupied may not feel like chatting. If you really want to talk to someone who might be busy, ask if he's available. "Have you got a minute?" It's like knocking to enter.

Recently Glenn started getting home from work an hour earlier. On the first day of the new schedule he looked forward to having a chance to talk with his sixteen-year-old son before dinner. He came in the door and called "Hi!" but there was no answer. Too bad, Jeremy must have stayed after school. But then a few minutes later, he heard Jeremy's radio playing upstairs.

Glenn climbed halfway up the stairs and called out, "Hey, Jeremy, it's me, Dad. Come on downstairs. I want to talk with you."

A few moments later Jeremy came into the living room and said, "What did I do?"

Glenn felt bad. Is that what their relationship had come to?

No, not really. Jeremy just felt off guard and misconstrued what his father meant. So now on days when he expects to be home early or wants to spend some time with Jeremy on the weekend, Glenn says something to him in the morning. "I'll be home around five-thirty. Maybe we can visit before supper."

• • •

Expectations about how and when communication should take place work not when they're right or wrong but when they're shared.

• • •

Self-Reflective Observation

Consideration for others helps make you sensitive enough to be a better listener. But even more important is developing self-reflective awareness. When you have trouble hearing someone or getting someone to hear you, step back and examine the process of communication between the two of you as just that—a *process*. You'll need to get beyond brooding about personalities to thinking about actions and reactions. And you'll need to get beyond the linearity of thinking that the other person *makes* you respond the way you do to seeing the process as circular.

Say that your teenage son never talks to you. Oh, he'll let you know when he needs new sneakers or a ride somewhere, but you miss the talks you used to have when he was younger. Now he's so sullen. You can write off this uncommunicativeness to adolescence if you like, or you can think of it as part of a circular process.

To reflect on your part in the process, ask yourself what might cause your son's reticence or what might reinforce it. Do you pry into things that teenagers keep private, like which of his friends smokes marijuana or drinks at parties? Do you bombard him with questions when he wants to retreat to the sanctuary of his room? And when he does open up, do you show respect for his opinions or argue with everything he says?

How Well Do You Listen to Yourself?

The respect for other people's feelings that makes you listen to them can be turned around to yourself. How well do you respect your right to think and feel what you do? How well do you listen to yourself?

Kate suffered from chronic headaches but had given up going to doctors because it never did any good. None of them ever figured out what was wrong, and few of them bothered to listen carefully to her complaints. Finally, at her sister's urging, she went to the headache clinic at a leading hospital in Boston.

One of the tests they did was a CAT scan of her brain. Afterward, Kate waited anxiously for the radiologist who would explain the results. When he finally arrived, it was clear that he was rushed. He introduced himself, but Kate didn't catch his name. Then he showed her the pictures from the CAT scan, and she saw a small white spot on the film. "That's just a normal calcification of your pineal gland," he said, "nothing to worry about."

As the doctor headed for the door, Kate felt unsatisfied and wished the conversation could have gone on a little longer. But she wasn't sure how to frame her questions and was embarrassed that she didn't remember the doctor's name.

Halfway out the door, the doctor turned and said, "Any other questions?"

Kate answered in a subdued voice, "No."

Kate heard the doctor's anxiousness to leave. But she was far less well tuned in to her own needs. Her fear and uncertainty, combined with the doctor's rushed manner, had created a cloud of fog surrounding her own needs.

● ● ●

**If you don't listen to yourself,
it's unlikely that anyone else will.**

● ● ●

Listening to yourself means not only respecting your own feelings but also getting to know something about your style of communicating. This isn't always easy, and it isn't always pleasant.

I, for example, have a penchant for making jokes and wisecracks in social situations. Maybe some of my jokes are funny, but they're often distracting. Joking around may be a defense against social anxiety, or maybe it's just an outlet for restless energy. Whatever the reasons for it, there are times when I have to make an effort to suppress the smart remarks that pop into my head.

You may find it easier to recognize other people's conversational habits you wish they would change. But the effort to understand your own ways will enable you to relate more effectively to other people, regardless of what they do.

In Chapter 2 I mentioned that one of the reasons people seek solitude is that they haven't learned to handle their anxiety around other people. But solitude has its uses. Being alone without distractions gives you time to listen to yourself. To hear your own thoughts. To think them through. Among the things you may find yourself thinking about are feelings you haven't been aware of and conversations that didn't go as well as you would have liked.

Most of us run around doing things all day. All too often, our actions are driven rather than undertaken with awareness. When you get caught up in a river of obligations, it winds up submerging your life as it carries you along.

"I Don't Have a Minute to Catch My Breath."

Well, here's your chance. Find a couple of times during the next few days to sit down with yourself without distractions. Tune in to your breathing. Concentrate on one full inhalation as it comes in and one exhalation as it goes out. One more in, and one more out. Relax and breathe. After you quiet down, listen to what's going on inside of you.

> Do you have the patience to wait till your mud settles and the water is clear?
>
> —LAO-TZU

I always regretted that I didn't go to a psychoanalytic institute after graduate school. So, after practicing for a number of years, I decided to go back and do it. At the institute I took classes and received supervision on my cases. In supervision you find out what you should have said, so that, hopefully, you'll do better next time. Supervision made me a better therapist, and it also made me feel a little stupid every week. *Why did I say that? Why didn't I see this?*

After finishing my course of study, I returned to my practice and became my own supervisor. I was by then much more aware after a session of things I missed or wished I had said. But instead of feeling stupid (or just feeling stupid), I started writing letters to patients between sessions. I might sum up what we talked about if I thought I hadn't made something clear, and sometimes I'd put things in the letter that I just hadn't thought of in the session.

Maybe you, too, are your own supervisor. Maybe you come away from certain conversations wishing you'd said something differently or wishing you'd been a better listener. You can try to do better next time, or you can seek out the person you have unfinished business with and try again to hear what he or she was saying and then clarify what you meant to say.

Exercises

1. Once or twice in the coming week, think about what you will be doing and whom you will be talking with. Predict what might happen if you made a concerted effort to listen to those people. Pick someone you care about. Consider what might distract you from listening. At the end of the day, take five minutes to reflect on what happened in those conversations. How well did you listen? What made it difficult? What was the result of your efforts?

2. Practice not interrupting people who are talking to you. Try to come up with two or three lines that invite people to finish what they're saying. You could say "mm-hmm," or "tell me more," or find something that seems to work for you. You may or may not find this device helpful. The point is not to interrupt. Cultivate patience.

3. Try asking "Do you have a minute?" before telling people what's on your mind. What effect does this seem to have on the quality of the listening you get?

9

• • •

"I Can See This Is Really Upsetting You"

How to Defuse Emotional Reactivity

We come now to the number-one reason people don't listen: reactive emotionalism. As we saw in Chapter 6, when someone says something that triggers anxiety, understanding goes out the window. If not acknowledging what the other person says turns discussions into conversational ping-pong, overreacting can turn them into the Battle of the Bulge. If the war metaphor seems melodramatic, take inventory of your feelings next time a series of attacks and counterattacks leaves you wounded.

Some people are so provocative that it's almost impossible to listen to them without getting upset. But regardless of what other people say, your problem is how you react.

And what about those thin-skinned individuals who fly off the handle at the slightest sign of criticism? Sure, they're overreactive, but unless your relationship to them is expendable, your challenge is finding a way to get through to them.

Empathy Turns Defensiveness Around

We're all insecure to some extent. Therefore, when we feel threatened, we tend to react defensively rather than being open to the other person's point of view.

One reason people pay thousands of dollars to psychotherapists is simply to be listened to. (Good therapists may do more than just listen, but they certainly do no less.) When people complain about other people in their lives, a therapist doesn't feel blamed and therefore doesn't get defensive. But when you talk to the people you're close to about your upsets, they feel implicated. That's why their response is often reactive: "No, don't feel that way!" An accepting, nonreactive response feels like "Yes, is that how you feel? Tell me more."

People Are Defensive for a Reason

When someone says, "You pay more attention to your parents than you do to me," a reactive response might be "I hardly ever see them!"

What imagined threat might the reactive partner be defending against?

What would be an empathic response to "You pay more attention to your parents than you do to me"?

How might an empathic response put you in a more vulnerable position? A more empowered position?

Empathy is permission giving. Receptive, nondefensive listeners allow us to get our feelings out. They welcome unpopular parts of us to speak (which allows us to do the same for ourselves). They recognize that even on those occasions when what we're saying about them may not be true, our feelings are.

• • •

Feelings are facts to the person experiencing them.

• • •

The simple—and often enormously difficult—act of not becoming reactive has a tremendous impact on relationships. It enables you to handle difficult conversations—and it empowers you to remain in control under pressure.

How to Avoid Reacting Emotionally When Provoked

Every so often Nadine lets out her frustration in the form of an emotional outburst about Tim's many failings:

"You're selfish and inconsiderate."

"You *never* think of anyone but yourself."

"You don't care about me; all you want is sex!"

Tim can't stand these tirades. *If she's unhappy, why can't she just say so without calling me every name in the book?* He tries to listen to her complaints, but by the time she's through dumping on him he just wants to go away and hide.

When Gordon complains about Jane's handling of the kids, she gets furious. First he leaves everything to her, then he criticizes her for doing what she thinks is right. *He's always right, and she's always wrong.* So she let's him know just how she feels.

All four of these people have a right to their feelings. The trouble is, no one is listening. To listen without flying off the handle, you have to learn to tolerate a certain amount of anxiety—and to resist the "fight or flight" urge.

"Don't Get Defensive!"

The trouble with this famous advice is that it's harder to stop doing something than it is to start doing something else. If you're trying to cut down on coffee, it's easier to pour yourself a cup of tea than to sit there not drinking coffee. If you want to stop eating junk food, it's easier to grab a carrot than to try to avoid the urge to rip open the potato chips. If you want to reduce your emotional reactivity, concentrate on listening harder.[1]

You probably know how it feels to be berated in an angry, assaultive way or found fault with by someone who's better at criticizing than helping. But getting reactive only makes things worse. Tim thinks his problem is Nadine's emotional exaggeration. But a fuller description of the problem would be that when Nadine feels ignored she tries not to say anything until she can't stand it anymore and then her feelings come pouring out— *and* Tim isn't able to pick up her signals of unhappiness before she explodes

---

[1] If "listening harder" seems abstract, just try listening longer.

or, when she does, to listen without getting angry and pulling away. Likewise, Jane's problem isn't just that Gordon leaves the children to her and then complains about her handling of them. Her reaction—getting mad and counterattacking—is part of what keeps Gordon from getting more involved. A full description of any listening problem must include both parties.

• • •

**What defeats us isn't the provocative speaker
but our own defensive response.**

• • •

The best way to master emotional reactivity is by having the courage to engage emotionally intense situations and tolerate the anxiety associated with that engagement. Avoiding such encounters affords only the illusion of self-control.

Ginny didn't call her mother after being in a car accident because she didn't want to have to deal with her mother's frantic questions and exaggerated concern. So she burdened herself with another secret and reinforced her own inability to deal with emotional pressure.

Learn to resist the impulse to act out your usual defensive response—avoiding, arguing, blaming, rebelling, dominating, or accommodating to achieve peace at any price. These reactions are driven by anxiety and designed to mask it by avoiding issues and defying, avoiding, or appeasing others. Facing up to people and situations you'd prefer to avoid, and learning to contain your own reactive reflexes, leads over time to a reduction of your anxiety.

In Chapter 6, I talked about hostile questions. Something a speaker says (or maybe it's just sitting there being lectured to) makes someone in the audience restive, and he or she attacks the speaker in the sublimated form of a question.

"Excuse me," said the eminent French deconstructionist Claude Nasal-Passages, who just happened to be in the audience, "but isn't everything you've just said total blather and you're full of nothing but helium?" In big words, of course.

Unfortunately, having just stood up in front of an audience for an hour or so pouring out their ideas, some speakers get a little touchy at such moments. And I've noticed (in other people, you understand) a certain unfortunate tendency to respond in kind.

"Well, yes, Professor Nasal-Passages, that's an intriguing point. But you're a pompous ass, and so is the horse you rode in on." Big words, again.

A better way to respond to hostile questions is to apply Formula Number One for resisting reactivity: hear the person out. Instead of agreeing or disagreeing, invite the questioner to say more. Hostile inquisitors aren't really asking questions; they just want to say something. So let them.

The same strategy works to keep reactivity from escalating in everyday conversations. Here's how a friend used this advice to reduce the antagonism that was starting to poison his second marriage.

When Rob married Carla, they got along wonderfully well except when it came to Rob's daughter. According to Carla, Rob spoiled Melanie, like lending her money and letting her have the car whenever she wanted, even though she didn't always bring it back when she said she would. But whenever Carla raised any objection, Rob felt she was attacking his child, and so instead of hearing what she had to say, he fought back. Many second marriages are broken on this very issue.

When Rob realized the situation had reached the point of crisis, he resolved to at least listen to Carla the next time she complained about Melanie. Two days later he got his chance. Melanie promised to have the car back by eight so Carla could go shopping, but she didn't get home until nine-thirty, after the stores were closed. When Carla complained to Rob, he felt his stomach knotting and the counterarguments forming. But instead of getting defensive, he said what he'd prepared himself to say: "Tell me more."

Carla said that overindulgence wasn't doing Melanie any good. Rob, sticking to his resolve not to interrupt, kept listening, and Carla went on. She talked about feeling like an outsider in her own house. She knew that Rob and Melanie had a special relationship, and she respected that. She had no wish to play Melanie's mother or tell Rob what to do. She just wanted to be able to talk to him when she felt concerned. Having determined not to argue, Rob found it remarkably easy to listen—that is, after he checked the rising emotions that Carla's first few sentences triggered in him. He stopped hearing in Carla the overbearing voice of his ex-wife, who was always so critical of the children, and started hearing how left out his new wife was feeling. He was able to hear that Carla wasn't asking him to change anything, just asking him to listen to her point of view. After that, things changed. They didn't always agree about how to respond to Melanie, but now that Rob knew that he could listen to Carla's opinion without necessarily following it, their differences ceased to divide them.

Prepare for Tense Encounters

The best way to defuse reactivity is to avoid becoming reactive yourself, something more easily said than done. One thing that helps is planning, as Rob was able to do once he realized how serious his breach with Carla was becoming. You can predict many of the difficult conversations in your life. If you stop to think about what the boss or your teenager is likely to say to trigger your anxiety, you can prepare for it.

● ● ●

Anticipation frees you from overreacting.

● ● ●

One way to remain calm is by schooling yourself to ask questions instead of flaring up at the usual provocations. This is a variation of the "tell me more" strategy. Another way to tone down emotionality is to respond to rhetorical questions and sarcasm literally, instead of being provoked into a defensive retort.

"Don't you ever think about anything but sex?"

"No, it's kind of a hobby with me. Like woodworking."

"Must you pick on every little thing I say?"

"Yes, all in the service of helping you become the perfect person I know you're capable of being."

How to Understand a Speaker's Anger

When people start to cry, we feel an urge to comfort them so that they'll stop. We equate the crying with pain. In fact, crying isn't pain; it's the way people release their pain. The same is true with expressions of anger (even if it's a little harder to keep that in mind).

I once watched a therapist interviewing a couple five years into a second marriage. They were having a hard time deciding how to balance their obligations to three sets of children and an even harder time keeping the discussion from turning into a shouting match. As the wife was saying her piece and starting to go on and on, rehashing the past and finding fault, her husband's foot started twitching ominously. Sitting behind the one-way mirror, I felt apprehensive. I could see an explosion coming but couldn't do anything about it.

Then the therapist, bless him, did exactly what needed to be done. He acknowledged what the wife had said and then let the husband speak— being careful to direct the husband's response to himself, who could listen, not to his wife, who at that point couldn't. Even so, the husband exploded. With hot emotion he refuted what his wife had said and explained the truth of things as he saw it. As he talked—with his wife blocked from responding—he calmed down perceptibly. His jaw relaxed, the tension went out of his shoulders, and his foot stopped twitching. Not having a chance to express his anger made it build. Expressing it, *even in an angry way*, released the anger.

The hard part would be teaching this couple to listen to each other without flying off the handle in the future. It's one thing to understand that expressing anger helps detoxify it; it's another thing to be on the receiving end.

The wife in the couple I observed was angry because her husband questioned her motives. She thought one of the children, who happened to be her son, needed some financial assistance. Her husband was jealous of the attention she paid this son and felt she was neglecting him. "He's twenty-three years old. He can take care of himself." But it wasn't disagreeing that caused their problems; it was getting reactive and shouting at each other. If he would concentrate on understanding what she was *feeling* and not allow himself to react defensively, he'd understand that she was worried about her boy. She might or might not decide to give him some money; that was just an idea, a way of expressing her concern. Her husband wasn't really upset about the money but about not getting as much attention as he used to. Unfortunately, instead of talking about his feelings, he blamed her for them.

• • •

**When feelings of not being understood come out as anger,
hearing them, not shutting your ears or fighting back,
is the key to calming things down.**

• • •

Kim knew she was in for it when she got home. Ernie expected her to tell him whenever she drove into the city, but she'd gone shopping without saying anything. She was going to be home before supper, but now she was stuck in traffic. As the cars crept along, her mind raced ahead.

Sure enough, when she walked into the house, Ernie demanded, "Where were you?"

"I had a little shopping to do at Macy's, and I got stuck in traffic."

"You didn't tell me you were going shopping."

She couldn't think of anything to say, so she said nothing.

Ernie went on about how he thought she'd agreed to tell him where she was going, and because she didn't have any excuse, Kim just listened.

It took less than two minutes for Ernie to finish complaining, and then he calmly went on to talk about other things.

Kim, who'd dreaded this confrontation, was amazed to discover that she didn't have to defend herself. All she had to do was listen.

Feelings don't always make sense right away. It's easier to hear feelings that don't come out as accusations, but if they do, remember that they are *feelings*, not scientific statements of fact. Don't yell back, call the other person names, or bring up old issues.

Denise was backing out of a parking space when she felt the SUV smack into the right side of her car. When she opened her door, the woman in the SUV was screaming at her. "Why don't you look where you're going, you stupid bitch!" Denise struggled to stay calm while she exchanged insurance information, called AAA, and rode to the garage in the tow truck. When she finally got home and told Henry what happened, she started to cry.

"That woman had no right to scream at me!" she said with rising emotion.

"Calm down," Henry said, "there's no reason to get upset. Just tell me what happened."

That's when Denise lost it. "Don't tell me to calm down!" she said.

"You're not the one whose car got smashed and then had to put up with that abuse!" At this point her anger shifted from that stupid woman to her husband's lack of sympathy.

• • •

Don't tell angry people to calm down. Doing so only makes them feel that you're denying their right to be upset.

• • •

If someone snaps at you in anger, how do you get beyond listening with a clenched mind? The obvious answer is to listen through the emotional static to what the person is trying to say. But that's easier said than done. When frustration and anger spill out into a relationship, our natural response is to become anxious and defensive. Listening to someone who assaults you with his feelings isn't easy. One thing that may help keep you from withdrawing into a defensive posture is hearing in the anxious speaker the voice of an unhappy child crying to be heard.

If, instead of dwelling on how difficult the speaker is, you can focus on your own efforts to listen and avoid overreacting, the anxiety in the relationship will begin to abate. Anxiety is electric. It requires conduction and amplification. If you listen and stay cool, the angry person will feel heard and begin to calm down.

In heated discussions, repeating the other person's position in your own words shows that you understand and interrupts your own defensive response. If the heat gets so intense that you start to seethe, try squeezing your thumb and index finger together. This momentary distraction (less hazardous to your health than "biting your tongue") may help you channel your tension in a way you can control.

If that doesn't work, or an emotionally reactive speaker is dumping on you and it's too upsetting, you may have to protest. Doing so before you get too upset, and without attacking, keeps your anger from boiling over: "I'm sorry, but I can't listen to this right now. I'm too upset. We'll have to talk later."

How to Take Criticism Without Overreacting

He says, "You're always late."

She says, "You're always rushing me."

One point for him. One point for her. Collective score: zero.

Allowing the other person to spell out his or her point of view before responding with yours is especially important—and especially difficult—when someone is criticizing you. If you start to react, ask yourself, Does the person have a sincere concern about this issue? If the answer is yes, keep listening.

If your spouse complains about where you park in the driveway, you might consider that he or she has a legitimate stake in the matter. If, on the other hand, he or she criticizes how you talk to your boss, you might remember that how you decide to talk to your boss is your business. Come to think of it, remembering that might make it easier to listen without feeling the need to defend yourself.

If someone criticizes you, stay with that concern; don't switch to a different criticism of your own. Avoid cross-complaining.

"Oh yeah? Well, what about you? You never take out the garbage when I ask you to."

"I don't care if you don't like what's for supper. Maybe if you cleaned up your room once in a while like I asked, I'd feel more like cooking something you like."

After you allow your critic to spell out his or her complaint, agree with whatever you can, or at least show appreciation for his or her concern.

"Yes, I have been a little grouchy lately. I'm sorry."

"So you think I've been favoring Cindy over Joshua?"

"Yes, I did run over your prize Pomeranian in the driveway. I'll get you a new one."

Okay, so I'm saying that when someone starts to criticize you, the thing to do is to hear him out and acknowledge his point of view before defending yourself. But isn't that a little like saying that to lose ten pounds all you have to do is cut out sweets? When someone starts in on you, especially someone close to you, it isn't easy to nod and say, "Oh, so you think I'm a selfish species of barnyard animal? I see. Please tell me more."

Listening to criticism is one of the hardest things we ever have to do. Unfortunately, getting defensive only makes things worse. To avoid doing so, train yourself to listen responsively—pay attention, appreciate what the other person is saying, and acknowledge it. This takes practice, but you can make it a habit. The active effort to listen helps prevent you from becoming reactive.

Focus on the issue. Try to hear in the criticism something the other person is asking you to do for him or her rather than a condemnation of yourself.

When Sid said, "I wish we didn't have to have fish every week," Nancy started complaining about how picky he was. "You're always complaining," she said. "For a while there you wouldn't eat meat; now that's *all* you want."

Sid was stung. He *never* complained about what Nancy cooked. He just hated the fish she served. *Didn't he have a right to say what he liked? Wasn't it better to be honest?* This kind of brooding internal dialogue is precisely what prevents us from appreciating the other person's point of view and fuels the likelihood of a reactive response.

If Sid could listen to Nancy for a minute, instead of to his own hurt feelings, he might realize that it's a big job figuring out what to serve for supper every night. Add in the complication of having to accommodate spouses' and children's preferences, and that those preferences change over time, and he might begin to understand what his wife was up against. If she expresses herself with "excessive" annoyance (Sid thinks: *All I said was I wish we didn't have to have fish*), that's a sign of stored-up resentment. Try to remember: expression *releases* resentment.

What if, despite all your efforts to be a patient listener, criticism comes out as an attack?

If criticism is given in a nasty or offensive way, you have a right to object to the manner in which the message was expressed. If you can't listen to someone who berates you in an assaultive way, simply state what put you off.

"I don't appreciate being called stupid" (or compared to my mother or called a bitch, or a son of one).

"I'll try to listen to your suggestion if you can say it in a less nasty way."

Actually, the word *nasty* is name-calling. Better to be concrete: "I'll try to listen to your suggestion if you can say it without telling me how selfish I am"—or "If you give me some idea of what you want instead of saying what a terrible person I am."

Will such remarks calm things down and allow the two of you to understand each other? Probably not. But sometimes you have to let other people know what your limits are.

"Why Does He [or She] Have to Talk Everything to Death?"

Jackie wishes twenty-four hours would go by without Fred's complaining about how nobody appreciates him at the office. Sometimes she feels like screaming. If he weren't so preoccupied with his precious career, maybe he'd get a little more appreciation from her and the children. She doesn't say so, of course. He'd only get mad and sulk. So whenever Fred starts in on topic number one, Jackie just sits there in pained silence.

Sam wishes Cheryl would stop launching into a diatribe every time she feels overwhelmed by taking care of the house and the kids. It isn't that she doesn't have a right to complain; it's the way she goes on and on about everything. He tries to be sympathetic, but it isn't easy. She'll say the house is a mess or the kids are awful, and then she'll just keep talking and talking, covering every little detail without ever really getting to the point. The worst of it, as far as Sam is concerned, is that she's always complaining about the same things. "'Suzie doesn't have any friends,' 'Suzie wasn't nice to so-and-so,' 'Suzie this,' 'Suzie that.' Why can't she leave the poor kid alone?"

The issues that come up over and over again represent people's core concerns. (*Their* core concerns, not necessarily your greatest shortcomings.) The more understood and accepted a person feels, the safer she feels to go deeper into these issues. The mechanical and repetitive feeling of some complaints stems partly from the fact that they rarely get a sympathetic hearing. Listening is the greatest gift you can give to help soothe a person's feelings. Fred's feeling that nobody appreciates his accomplishments and Cheryl's worries about the children will never be completely resolved. That's why they need to talk about these things from time to time.

When people bring up recurring issues, some of us get upset and say something like "How many times do we have to go through this?" Such retorts make sense if you feel that the speaker's complaints mean that you're responsible or that it's your job to solve whatever problem the person is complaining about. But is it really your job to resolve your mother's complaints about your sister or your mate's complaints about the children? Once you understand that other people's talking about what's bothering them makes them feel better, you can relax, knowing that just listening without becoming reactive can make both of you feel better.

• • •

Sharing problems makes people feel understood.
Listening is how we help them feel better
and how we build closer relationships.

• • •

For those who can get beyond blaming others for "making" them upset, discovering what triggers their sensitivity leads to the question "Where does my emotional reactivity come from?"

Getting to the Root of Reactivity

Reactivity develops as a defense against personal attacks. The more our parents listened, took us seriously, and respected our opinions and feelings, the more secure and self-possessed we became. The less they listened, the more intolerant and critical they were, the more insecure and anxious we became. The more exposed we were to accusations and arguments, the more we learned to become defensive.

What happens in your family when people get anxious? Do they get into shouting matches? Stop talking and avoid each other? That's your legacy.

Back to the Past

Making peace with your parents means being in emotional contact with them, being yourself, and letting them be themselves. Changing your relationship to them doesn't mean changing them; it means changing the

---

way you react to them. Notice what they do that drives you crazy. Notice how you respond. *That* you can change. The more you learn to resist the urge to flare up in the face of their provocations, the more self-possessed and unflappable you'll become in all the rest of your relationships. When it comes to emotional reactivity, your parents are the final exam.

Remember Peggy from Chapter 5? She was the woman whose mother's negativism provoked her into shouting matches. Peggy learned to see how her mother's negativism triggered her own rage—and how expecting it made her hypersensitive. Seeing this pattern was one thing; changing it was another.

When Peggy decided to stop trying to change her mother, she began to realize that her mother wasn't really a mean person, just someone who prized togetherness so much that she was threatened when people acted independently. This simple shift in Peggy's view of her mother made it a lot easier for her to listen the next time she heard her mother criticizing someone in the family for doing something different. However, she also found that simply remaining silent only made her seethe. So instead of just holding her tongue or criticizing her mother (for being critical!) she started to say, as calmly as possible, that she could see how her mother saw it but she didn't agree.

At first Peggy's effort to clarify where she stood, rather than criticize her mother, was lost on her mother. "Oh, so you think I'm all wrong, do you?"

Much to Peggy's credit, she was able to maintain a calm, nonreactive position, even if her insides were churning. She listened until her mother was through and didn't contradict her or fight back.

When Peggy finally did speak, she said, "No, Mom, you're not hearing me. I'm not saying you're all wrong. I don't think that at all. You have a right to your opinion. I'm just saying that my opinion is different, that's all."

In the ensuing months, as Peggy continued to make an effort to speak up calmly when she disagreed with her mother's uncharitable opinions, she tried to make it clear that she was declaring her independence but not any lack of love or respect. On the contrary, as she learned to overcome her inability to tolerate her mother's criticism, the two women began to get closer. Peggy still occasionally slipped back into blaming and distancing, but not for long, and when this happened, instead of thinking of her mother as impossible and herself as helpless, she realized that she was just getting reactive again. That made it easier to control.

She and her mother still argued from time to time, but now Peggy spoke up before her annoyance reached the boiling point. That and the fact that instead of criticizing her mother she made a point of simply clarifying where she stood made the arguments much less toxic.

After things calmed down between her and her mother, Peggy decided to work on her relationship with her father. Growing up, she'd thought of him as distant and unapproachable, a large and benevolent shadow at the edge of the family circle. She remembered him sitting silently behind the newspaper while she and her mother fixed dinner or chatted at the breakfast table. Now she longed to be closer to him but didn't know how to go about it. How do you talk to a shadow? After she'd married and had children, she made a concerted effort to get closer to him. He'd listen politely when she told him about the children's latest doings, but as soon as she said anything about her job or her friends, his eyes would drift in the direction of the television, or he'd suddenly remember something he had to do. As far as Peggy was concerned, he might as well have slapped her in the face.

What Peggy felt as rejection from her father was in fact anxiety about intimacy. Her efforts to get closer to him took the form of pursuing a distancer, a pattern she also played out with her husband.

Intimacy has levels of intensity, from simple contact, to chatting about neutral subjects like the weather, to semipersonal topics, to personal conversations about things that are important to you, to talking about your relationship. Everyone gets anxious at some point on this progression; precisely where depends on you and who you're with. Peggy's father just happened to be one of those people made anxious by even mildly intimate conversations. It wasn't that he didn't love his daughter; he just didn't know how to talk to her.

To get closer to her father, I advised Peggy to spend a little time alone with him—which meant gently pulling him out of hiding behind the television—and away from the grandchildren—and moving the conversation very slowly from one level of intimacy to the next, stopping as soon as either one of them started to get anxious. Pushing her father past his comfort zone would only trigger his distancing reflex and leave Peggy feeling like a fisherman after the big one got away.

Peggy lowered her expectations and decided simply to spend some time with her father, during which she would keep the conversation light. Her primary concern would be to avoid becoming anxious or making her father feel that way. She found her father remarkably receptive to this new nondemanding approach and on her next visit hoped to move the conversation to a slightly more personal level.

She had complained that her father showed no interest in her life, but now she realized that she hadn't demonstrated much interest in his. I suggested that she try an opening that most people will respond to: "What are you working on these days?" Peggy's father welcomed his daughter's interest, and he reciprocated by showing more interest in what was going on in her world. Once or twice when she tried to talk about something that made her father uncomfortable—like how his retirement money was holding out—he did his old disappearing act, and Peggy once again felt rejected. But she didn't dwell on this feeling, and it didn't last long. Her father never did become the kind of man she could really confide in, but he was after all her father, and she loved him. What's more, now that she'd come to terms with his reticence, she realized how much he loved her.

"I've Tried to Change Things with My Parents, but It Hasn't Worked."

Systems are tenacious, resistant to change; or to put it in more human terms, your parents have a long history of relating to you in a certain way. If you try to change that, you will be tense and their reaction will be intense. Have a plan when you visit. Remember that when you reenter the family's emotional force field, your ability to think about what's going on is impaired. So do your thinking beforehand. Formulate reasonable goals. When you try a new way of behaving, start with small steps.

The people close to us don't have any tricks up their sleeves. Their actions surprise us only because we keep looking for them to do what we wish they'd do. They do what they do. Once you learn this, you can stop being surprised and upset. You can let them be who they are. You might as well; they will anyway.[2]

A relationship matures when you can allow the other person to be who he or she is. If your mother criticizes everybody *and* you can't accept this, your life may be dominated by your attempt to stop her (and everybody else, for that matter) from criticizing anything or anyone. Once you can let your mother be a person who's critical—in other words, accept that she is who she is—you don't have to fight it or organize your life around it.

• • •

Once you accept that people are who they are,
you can stop trying to change them—and stop overreacting
when they do *what they've always done*.

• • •

Peggy's more relaxed approach to her parents didn't stop her mother from being critical or her father from being withdrawn, but it did make Peggy a whole lot less reactive to them—and to the other people in her life who touched the same raw nerves.

Learning to listen without overreacting is an exercise in accepting that each of us is different and separate. You can even learn to enjoy the differences. Formerly "difficult" and "disagreeable" people begin to soften perceptibly as soon as you let them be who they are.

Why Emotional Reactivity Increases
as Relationships Evolve

In the early stages, most relationships are fairly comfortable. People can talk and listen without too much tension; otherwise the relationship wouldn't get very far. Such harmony, however, is time-limited. Relationships, like unstable chemical compounds, tend to deteriorate. Once a relationship becomes heated with emotional reactivity, it may have to be cooled down with emotional distance—avoidance of one another or at least of potentially upsetting subjects. But if the two parties are closeted together or try

---

[2]One of my patients once told me without irony that her father "could be a wonderful person, if only he were different."

to discuss emotionally charged issues, one or both of them may start spilling over with anxiety.

One person may act to preserve harmony by giving in and doing all the listening. The other person may be unaware of the disparity. But it takes two to preserve this inequality. The mistake the placater makes is to confuse self-denial with self-restraint. The latter strategy allows both people to win; the former makes losers of them both. But as long as one person is cowed by the other's emotionality, and the other continues to express himself in the same old way, both of them are preserving the unhappy equilibrium.

The emotional climate in a relationship varies from hot to cold, turbulent to stable, and safe to unsafe. The presence of unresolved conflict makes for storminess. Some relationships, for example, are dominated by friction over togetherness versus independence. Anything said about who's going to do what with whom can trigger the anxiety over this conflict.

When someone opens up on you with a mean mouth or listens with only feigned interest, it's natural to blame his or her personality. When someone erupts at something you say, it's impossible not to blame this outburst on him or her. But reactivity, like everything else in a relationship, is interactional. The only part of the equation you can change is your part.

● ● ●

**Trying to avoid or control other people
doesn't resolve your reactivity.**

● ● ●

A listener's oversensitivity festers and flourishes with preoccupation about giving too much or getting too little. Unfortunately, this listener's reactivity makes people avoid him or her, which increases the listener's alienation and exacerbates his or her reactivity. As their emotional composure decreases, people rely more on other people to provide their sense of well-being. This dependence inflates expectations and escalates reactivity.

● ● ●

**To cut down on reactivity, respect your right to be yourself
and other people's right to be themselves.**

● ● ●

Self-possessed people aren't easily threatened by loss of their own emotional integrity, and so their relationships are flexible. Periods of closeness and distance are tolerated. Each is free to be close or pursue their own interests. Neither is threatened by the other's needs. Denying one's own emotional reactions, blaming those reactions on others, and avoiding or pursuing others to reduce anxiety are emotionally driven processes that rob relationships of flexibility. The point isn't to deny your feelings but to choose how to react to them.

Mature listeners take responsibility for their own responses. Instead of thinking "So and so is impossible," they hear what is said, feel their reactions, and then decide how to respond.

"Hearing" someone who doesn't open up means recognizing that he doesn't want to say much. If the reticent person is someone you care about, you may feel shut out. But if you react to that feeling by pressuring the other person to open up, you are projecting your own anxiety and making him or her feel threatened.

Pressuring someone to open up isn't listening. You may really want to hear what's on his mind, you may think you can help, you may believe it would be good for him and the relationship if he talked more; but pressure is pressure.

The best way to approach emotionally reticent people is to make contact without pushing. Openness without pressure helps relax the assumption that it isn't safe to open up. Respecting the integrity of the emotional boundary that allows you to be yourself (someone who wants to get closer) and the other person to be himself or herself (someone who wants to go slow) keeps anxiety from escalating.

Releasing yourself from slavish and unrewarding obligations helps stem the energy drain from a few expendable relationships. But since most of our relationships aren't expendable, the most important thing you can do to avoid getting caught up in emotionally reactive transactions is to stay calm and be yourself. Staying open means honoring other people's individuality; staying receptive means not denying your own.

● ● ●

The self-possessed listener is not isolated or unfeeling but nonreactive.

● ● ●

How to Tone Down Your Message and Be Heard

You know how frustrating it is not to be listened to. But how often do you stop to consider that there might be something about the way you express yourself that makes others deaf to your concerns?

Several years ago my friend John tried to teach me how to tune up my temperamental English motorcycle. When he showed up on the appointed day and saw how nervous I was, he said, "The first thing you have to do is calm down." How do you calm down when you're about to take apart a fifteen-thousand-dollar piece of machinery on which you'll later be going over a hundred miles an hour? But he was right. The way my hands were shaking I'd never have been able to shim the diphthongs with the krenging hook. So we repaired to the kitchen for a beer. Later I had the satisfaction of knowing that it wasn't getting all wound up that made me unable to put the damn thing back together. It's just that I'm a natural born klutz.

Why is it that when it comes to relationship problems so few of us bother to follow my friend John's advice and calm down before we start?

As we've seen, one way speakers undermine their messages is to say things with such anger and upset that the listener becomes so anxious that he or she doesn't clearly register—and therefore doesn't remember—the content of the speaker's message. All that gets communicated is the upset. Suppose, for example, that once every few months a wife gets so tired of her husband's always leaving the bathroom a mess that she blows up about it. It infuriates her that he doesn't remember—even after she's told him how upset it makes her. All he remembers is getting yelled at.

It's hard to listen when you feel attacked. That's why even though you may have complained about something for years, other people never really get it. You've told them a million times; still they don't understand. Anxiety is the enemy of listening.

One message sure to give someone's hackles a workout is pointing out financial extravagances. Here's the great humorist S. J. Perelman illustrating his technique.

Weary of pub-crawling and eager to recapture the zest of courtship, we had stayed home to leaf over our library of bills, many of them first editions. As always, it was chock-full of delicious surprises: overdrafts, modistes' and milliners' statements my cosset had concealed from me, charge accounts unpaid since the Crusades. If I felt any vexation, however, I was far too cunning to admit it. Instead, I turned my pockets inside out to feign insolvency, smote my forehead distractedly in the tradition of the Yiddish theater, and quoted terse abstracts from the bankruptcy laws. But fiendish feminine intuition was not slow to divine my true feelings. Just as I had uncovered a bill from Hattie Carnegie for a brocaded bungalow apron and was brandishing it under her nose, my wife suddenly turned pettish.

"Sixteen dollars!" I was screaming. "Gold lamé you need yet! Who do you think you are, Catherine of Aragon? Why don't you rip up the foyer and pave it in malachite?" With a single dramatic gesture, I rent open my shirt. "Go ahead!" I shouted. "Milk me—drain me dry! Marshalsea prison! A pauper's grave!"

"Ease off before you perforate your ulcer," she enjoined. "You're waking the children."

"You think sixteen dollars grows on trees?" I pleaded, seeking to arouse in her some elementary sense of shame.[3]

Notice how Perelman employs his knowledge of psychology. Shaming someone is a sure way to get her attention.

Here's Perelman demonstrating how to handle the delicate subject of gratuities. He and his family are moving out of their apartment, and he's faced with the challenge of appropriately expressing his gratitude for the staff's service.

Heaped by the curb were fourteen pieces of baggage exclusive of trunks; in the background, like figures in an antique frieze, stood the janitor, the handyman, and the elevator operators, their palms mutely extended. I could see that they were too choked with emotion to speak, these men who I know not at what cost to themselves had labored to withhold steam from us and jam our dumbwaiters with refuse. Finally one grizzled veteran, bolder than his fellows, stepped forward with an obsequious tug at his forelock.

"We won't forget this day, sir," the honest chap said, twisting his cap in his gnarled hands. "Will we, mates?" A low growl of assent ran round the circle. "Many's the time we've carried you through that lobby and a reek of juniper off you a man could smell five miles down wind. We've seen some strange sights in this house and we've handled some spectacular creeps; it's kind of like a microcosm like, you might say. But we want you to know that never, not even in the nitrate fields of Chile, the smelters of Nevada, or the sweatshops of the teeming East Side, has there been a man—" His voice broke off and I stopped him gently.

"Friends," I said huskily, "I'm not rich in worldly goods, but let me say this—what little I have is mine. If you ever need anything, whether jewels,

---

[3]S. J. Perelman, *The Swiss Family Perelman* (New York: Simon & Schuster, 1950), pp. 4–5.

money, or negotiable securities, remember these words: you're barking up the wrong tree. Geronimo."[4]

Notice that even though Perelman's message might have been a trifle unwelcome, his delivering it calmly enabled him to drive off to a chorus of ringing cheers (or so it seemed from a distance).

But seriously, folks, what can you do when someone becomes reactive? Perhaps whenever you say anything the least bit critical, a certain someone gets angry and shuts down. Try getting less invested in being heard but remain open to the relationship on the other person's terms. This can be done without compromising yourself. It's the difference between self-denial—caving in—and self-restraint—waiting for your turn.

Say, for example, that whenever a wife tells her husband, even very nicely, that he shouldn't put certain dishes in the dishwasher, he gets that wounded look and withdraws into hurt silence. The same thing happens when she complains about his not making the household repairs he's promised: he sulks. She feels like she's living with a big baby. But if she can calm down enough to ask herself where her criticism comes from, she might discover that it stems from unrealistic expectations.

The people you live with have assets and limitations. If you pitch your expectations at their assets instead of their limitations, you stand a better chance of being heard. Coming to terms with the real person you're relating to, rather than agonizing over the fact that he or she isn't different, will do a lot to lower your reactivity.

Learn what makes people reactive and try to defuse it with preparatory comments.

"I'm not saying it's your fault, but I'm tired of seeing the kids leave their toys all over the place."

"I'm not sure how to say this … "

If you're trying to make a request, not an attack, say so. But maybe you should examine your motives a little more carefully. When you say the kids shouldn't leave their toys around, do you really feel that it's your partner's fault for allowing it? Is the inference he or she reacts to accurate? Even if you don't make such criticisms explicit, they often come through.

---

[4]Perelman, pp. 16–17.

If you want someone to hear what you have to say without getting into a snit, don't forget tone and timing. Do you bring things up at the wrong time? Do you allow a judgmental tone to creep into your voice?

If someone you know gets annoyed when you offer advice, inquire before doing so. "Would you like some advice, or would you rather I just listen?" If you intend to bring up an upsetting subject, give a warning. What makes something traumatic is being overwhelmed. A person who isn't prepared is more easily overwhelmed. The more reactivity you anticipate, the more important it is to set the scene. A note or phone call telling someone you need to talk to them about something will help him gird himself.

• • •

Although it may seem artificial, putting difficult messages in notes is an effective way to short-circuit reactivity.

• • •

Ultimately, of course, it isn't other people's overreaction that's your problem but how *you* react to that. You don't have to get upset when someone else does.

One thing to remember when emotional reactivity drowns out listening is that *it's always your move.* Waiting for other people to change—or hammering at them in hopes that they will—is understandable but unproductive. Sometimes it makes sense to write off unrewarding relationships that aren't central to your life. The person who's so touchy that anything you say can trigger an angry response may be more trouble than he or she is worth. Unfortunately, some of us are more likely to give up on relationships that *are* central to our lives—spouses, parents, colleagues—because they're the hardest to manage.

"What's Wrong with Him?"

The next time someone overreacts to what you're saying, ask yourself, "Where does this emotional response come from?" "What sore spot must I have touched?" rather than "What's wrong with him or her?"

The following remarks add fuel to the fire:

"You're such a baby!"

"Someone got up on the wrong side of the bed today!"

"Can't you take a simple suggestion?"

"You sound just like your mother."

"You're so immature."

"Is it that time of the month again?"

"What's eating you? Every time I open my mouth you bite my head off."

According to Claire, her son Jeffrey is oversensitive. The least little thing she says to him can make him fly into a rage. One time she told him that his teacher probably wouldn't pick on him so much if he acted more mature in class, and he burst into tears and ran into his room. "He's always throwing tantrums," Claire said.

A child who bursts into tears and runs out of the room isn't throwing a tantrum. Kids aren't stupid. If they pitch a fit because they want to bend you to their wishes, they do it in front of you. (If you want to defuse a temper tantrum, remove the audience.)

The way to resolve reactivity is to understand it, not judge it. Imagine a little boy storming out of the room after his mother said something to him. Why would a child get so upset? Often it's because what she said made him feel shamed. When someone feels humiliated, he becomes foot-stompingly outraged; he is I-am-wronged! Injuries to self-respect are as bruising as muggings. If you asked him what was wrong, he'd probably say "Mommy yelled at me" or perhaps "Nothing, leave me alone!"

Few of us, children least of all, label our experience as shame. Unfortunately, parents who don't recognize a shame reaction or can't tolerate a child's upset get into a tug of war that makes things worse. They demand to know what's wrong, as if a child convulsed with emotion could say.

Give a shamed person room to hide and lick his wounds. Shame is so painful that the child momentarily loses control of his feelings. He needs time to regain his composure. Let him have it.

If someone becomes enraged at something you said, think about how you might have offended his dignity. Did you treat him like a baby? Imply that his opinion was invalid? That his feelings aren't legitimate? The way to decode an "excessive" emotional response isn't to blame the other person—or yourself—but to consider what the exposed nerve might be.

Sometimes It's a Mistake to Try to Control Your Feelings

Some people are afraid to speak at funerals or weddings because they might start to cry—as if crying were a sign of weakness, not compassion. "But," one woman protested when I tried to tell her there's nothing wrong with crying, "if I start to cry, I won't be able to finish what I want to say."

If you start to cry and tell yourself that's awful and try to stop, you may well have trouble speaking. It's hard to concentrate on two things at once. But if your heart moves and your feelings show, what's wrong with that?

A trick some people use to help them cope with their anxiety about public speaking is to accept rather than fight their nervousness. "Good morning. My name is so-and-so, and I'm a little nervous speaking in front of such a large group." Such candor makes listeners sympathetic. Most of us know what it feels like to be nervous speaking in public. Even more important, though, is the effort to accept your feelings as natural instead of trying to fight them.[5]

There's an even more important way that trying to resist feelings leads to more reactivity. If you let someone know how angry you are by venting your bottled-up frustration in an emotional outburst, you're likely to come across as attacking. If the other person responds with angry counteraccusations or just walks out, you may conclude that it was a mistake to talk about your feelings. This conclusion leads to a control and release cycle. You hold everything in until you explode. The solution isn't more control but less.

• • •

Speaking up sooner makes it easier to lower your voice.

• • •

Instead of "You never do anything around here," try "I'm overloaded with housework. I need more help."

Don't turn discussions into a *zero-sum game*, in which one person wins (is right) only if the other loses (is wrong).

There is, however, a difference between expressing what you feel and dumping your emotions. Recently I got into an argument with a woman

---

[5]Thinking about "communicating with people" instead of "speaking in front of them" will shift your attention and help you calm down.

who was tired of her father-in-law's belittling comments and planned to tell him off. When I suggested she tone down her emotionality before talking to him, she blew up at me. "What's wrong with getting angry?" she demanded.

This woman had a reason to be angry. Her father-in-law's cutting remarks were hard to take. But if she allowed her upset to overwhelm her, her complaints wouldn't be voiced clearly and wouldn't be heard. Unloading her anger, rather than articulating her complaints, would allow her father-in-law to dismiss her as "oversensitive" or "having a bad day." I'm not advocating emotional detachment. Anger helps preserve our integrity and self-regard, but simply venting anger doesn't usually solve the problem it signals. The distinction I'm trying to draw isn't between emotion and reason but between impulsive and deliberate action. There's nothing wrong with emotion, and there's nothing wrong with telling someone off, if that's what you want to do. It's not responding with feeling that makes us feel childish and inept—it's losing control.

Exercises

1. For a week, keep track of the number of your communications that are (a) critical or instructional, (b) avoidant, or (c) affectionate or laudatory. To change the climate in a relationship, shift from (a) and (b) to (c) and see what happens.

   This deceptively simple exercise may be very difficult to do. But trying it may help you begin to think more about how you're coming across to the people you care about.

2. What kind of interactions make you lose your cool? Do you have trouble with anger? Do you start to cry when you talk about your feelings? Do you get flustered in arguments?

   Find a reasonably safe occasion in the next week or so when you can put yourself in a situation you usually become reactive in. For example, if you have teenagers, you can predict that they're likely to test the limits of house rules; if you have little ones, you can expect them to ask for treats. One of the easiest ways to identify situations that make you reactive is to think about what situations you habitually avoid. Don't expect too much of yourself, just concentrate on getting through the experience without losing your cool. (Hint: One way to avoid losing your cool is to focus on drawing the other person out.)

3. The next time someone overreacts, consider where that reaction might be coming from. If you can do this during a confrontation, you're a better person than I am. But you can always think about a blowup later. You get an A+ on this assignment if you can use that sensitivity to express empathy for what the other person seems to be feeling. (Remember: you can always seek the person out and make amends later.)

4. You probably know people who could use some of the suggestions in this chapter. Why not buy several additional copies of this book and leave them scattered around in strategic places?

Part Four

· · ·

Listening in Context

10

. . .

"We Never Talk Anymore"

Listening Between Intimate Partners

It started innocently enough. She met him at an office party and all they did was talk. But when Maureen got home and her husband asked if she had a nice time, she found herself unwilling to mention Arthur, as though he were a secret she didn't want to lose by telling. The next day Arthur called to invite her for lunch. One lunch followed another, and then there were drinks after work. The following week they drove up to Thatcher Park and talked as they watched the sun set over the valley below. Nothing happened, unless you count the brief moment when Maureen's glance left Arthur's eyes and dropped to his lips and a shiver ran through her.

It was at this point that Maureen consulted me. She felt on the brink of something. Arthur was everything her husband wasn't: successful, self-possessed, but most of all he really listened when they talked. Telling me this, Maureen was visibly nervous. Her eyes scanned mine, looking for understanding, expecting perhaps judgment, or maybe permission to do what she longed to.

When, I asked, did the passion in her marriage die? She looked away. Then she wiped her eyes and said that her husband was a good person; they'd just ... grown apart. He never talked to her anymore.

My sympathies were with this woman. Life holds few choices as consequential as the one between satisfaction and security. Still, I'd seen too many stale marriages blamed on the other partner.

When I suggested she bring her husband to our second meeting, Maureen was reluctant. She wasn't looking for marital therapy, she said, and she was afraid of Raymond's finding out about Arthur. What finally overcame her hesitation was her hope that if I saw what Raymond was like, maybe I'd understand why she'd consider leaving him.

Raymond did come, and Maureen told him she was unhappy with their marriage. He seemed sympathetic, as though accustomed to obliging, but not really engaged. He listened but didn't say much. Only when I asked about his work did Raymond become animated. We talked for a few minutes until Maureen interrupted to complain that he never talked to her about these things. Why couldn't he share his feelings with her? Raymond didn't have a very good answer for that. I was encouraged. Here was something to work on.

If two people can't talk, I said, something's wrong. Then I turned their chairs to face each other and asked Raymond to talk to Maureen about his work and what his concerns were. I told her to listen and help him bring out his feelings.

Raymond talked about the anxieties of opening a new law practice in the middle of a recession. Very little work was coming in, but he was convinced that if he could hang on for another year or so, things would start to turn around. Maureen broke in to say that things would never improve until he got rid of that idiot Ernie, his partner. They argued for a minute, and then Raymond shut up.

Here was one reason this couple didn't talk. When Raymond talked about what was on his mind, Maureen argued or advised; he protested feebly, then folded his tent. Perhaps she was comfortable with conversational give-and-take and he wasn't. Maybe he couldn't listen to her opinions because he didn't believe in his own power to decide what to do. In any case, here was a concrete problem to address.

Before I could start to help these two sort out their relationship, I had to talk privately with Maureen. I would propose a trial nonseparation, a period of not seeing Arthur and putting her energy into improving the marriage, so she could find out if it could be improved.

Maureen was relieved that I'd met Raymond. "Now you see," she said, "how bad our relationship is. It's never going to change." (Maureen was a great believer in chemistry, that famous force of attraction with more power to excite than endure.) Nothing I said about postponing any decision until she'd waited a few weeks to see if the marriage could be improved made any impact. She started seeing Arthur again that same week, and when Raymond found out the following week, he was as forgiving as most husbands.

Their divorce was finalized a year and a day after the one time I saw them together, eleven months after Maureen's affair with Arthur heated up, and eight months after it ended. Maureen was left with the house, two children, mortgage payments she couldn't keep up with, and the memory of that shiver.

Maureen viewed her marriage as a predicament, an entity, something with a history, perhaps, but one that after a while takes on a life of its own. Most of us feel this way at times. But a relationship is not a thing, not a static state; it is a process of mutual influence. A relationship isn't something you have; it's something you do.

● ● ●

**Couples who learn to listen to each other—
with understanding and tolerance—often find that
they don't need to change each other.**

● ● ●

The impulse to change things, to make them better, is a natural and largely constructive one. But anyone who thinks of marriage as an infinitely improvable arrangement is making a mistake. The ideal of perfectibility breeds frustration. Many problems can be solved, but the problem of living with another person who doesn't always see things the way you do isn't one of them. Sometimes marriage isn't about resolving differences but learning to live together with them.

What Goes Around

When I was in the third grade, Miss Halloway used a stroboscope to show us how light affects what we see. Late one winter afternoon when the shadows were long she took out a small fan with a metal blade and plugged it in. She turned on the switch, and the blade began to spin and then whir. Then she turned on the stroboscope. As she adjusted the rate of flash, the fan blade slowed down and then stopped. The blade looked so still and harmless! How easy it would be, I thought, to reach out and touch it.

The blade looks stationary, Miss Halloway explained, because the stroboscope illuminates only one point in the cycle. As I came to realize later, this is the same way we see our relationships.

The first thing to understand about couples is that *complementarity* is the governing principle of relationship. Behavior doesn't take place in a vacuum but in the context of relationships in which we act and react to each other. In any relationship, one person's behavior is functionally related to the other's. If at times we see only one point in the cycle—a friend's failure to call, for example, or a partner's lack of interest in what we have to say—that doesn't mean that relationships don't spin around in a circle.

The greatest impediment to understanding in intimate relationships is the injured feeling of unfairness that makes us look outside ourselves for the sources of our disappointment. We can't help wishing our mates would be a little more interested in what we have to say and a little less defensive about what we have to say about them. At about this time, the romantic vision of marriage gives way to melodrama—the story of villain and victim that unhappily married people tell themselves and, when things get bad enough, anyone else who will listen.

Many couples expect too much of each other and see their difficulties as more apocalyptic than they really are. The real tragedy of this tragic view is that our ability to see what's going on is compromised. Like Maureen, we fix on the hurtful things our partners do and think of our troubles as inevitable.

When all is said and done, marriage and its famous complications can be illuminated by focusing on one thing: the basic pattern of interaction between two people. Start with the hurtful things your partner does—the avoidance or selfishness or irritability—but then ask yourself: What is the complementary other half of this pattern?

It Takes Two to Tango

Whenever you have a problem with someone, note what the person does that bothers you; then consider what the other half of that pattern might be. This might just give you the key to unlocking the problem.

Complaint	Complement
"He doesn't talk to me."	He doesn't like the way you listen.
"She's not very affectionate."	She has unspoken resentments.
"He's selfish."	He thinks you're selfish.
"He never asks me how my day went."	You never ask him how his day went.

The other half of the equation—your part—doesn't have to be something you do that causes the problem. It might just be your way of keeping it going.

What Annoys You	What Perpetuates It
"He touches me in a way I don't like."	You don't show him how you like to be touched.
He thinks "Here we go again."	He never lets you get to the heart of your concerns and makes you feel that he understands.

Rhythms of Change in a Committed Relationship

Although the cycle of human life may be orderly, it isn't a steady, continuous march. Periods of growth and change are followed by times of relative stability in which changes are consolidated. The good news is that life isn't one long uphill struggle; sometimes you reach a plateau and can coast. The bad news is that you can't stay forever in one place. Partnership, too, has its cycles and seasons.

Courtship—what a lovely, old-fashioned word—is a time of opening up and testing for compatibility. Enchanted by romance, the partners are absorbed and engaged with each other. Conversation flows, and listening comes easily. They find each other so novel and delightful. So attentive, so interesting, so *interested*.

Fascination makes them overlook gaps in listening. Something puts her in mind of high school, and she asks him what it was like for him. He reminisces fondly about his experience, but when he doesn't reciprocate, doesn't ask her what it was like for her, she thinks it's an oversight. She'll get her turn later.

Young and in love, we take such pleasure in each other's company that sober considerations give way to dictates of the heart. Falling in love is an act of imaginative creation. Later, our hearts may shrink, and with it our eagerness to listen. But that's later. Now, although we might be more compatible with partners more like ourselves, nature's urge to mix genes draws us to the otherness of the other.

• • •

The great challenge of courtship is to come together and still be yourself.

• • •

With love at stake, we lie a little. We tell tender lies, a few self-protecting lies, and more than a few self-deluding lies. Looking back, we wish we'd been more honest, hadn't tried so hard to get our partners to like us.

When courting couples move in the direction of their intentions, trying to discover how far they can go together, it's usually two steps forward and one step back. Over the years a dozen or so couples have sought me out for premarital counseling. What a good idea, I used to think. Unfortunately, these encounters often turn out to be quite frustrating. The people seeking help come not because they are amazingly cautious but because they are amazingly mismatched. Despite that, most of them have passed an emotional point of no return and intend to marry, no matter what. Among the obstacles they will overcome is their own good judgment.

• • •

If courtship were more conscious, people would pay more attention to the quality of one another's listening.

• • •

Among the most important things to find in a mate is someone who's easy to talk to. Making friends and being able to talk to each other is a far more reliable guide than good looks, cleverness, or that dizzy feeling that people call "falling in love." (Try telling that to someone in love.)

He Needs Space; She Wants Closeness[1]

He wants to be left alone and she wants attention. So she gives him attention and he leaves her alone.

Jack and Irene were a handsome couple, in their mid-thirties. Irene was a pretty woman, with ash-blond hair and an energetic look. The day they came to see me she was wearing a linen suit with a silk blouse. Jack, tall and slender, wore jeans. She'd dressed up; he'd dressed down. Was it just a different approach to this interview or a different approach to life?

"What brings you to therapy?" I asked, looking at both of them.

Jack answered first. "Well, I'm a little intolerant."

"What does Irene do that's hard to tolerate?"

They exchanged looks. Irene gave Jack a faint smile, and he turned back to me. "She yammers. She makes assumptions, and there's nothing I can do about it—about what she assumes—so I give up and go on about my business."

"You mean, you pull away?"

"Well ... yes."

He went on to describe himself as a man who isn't very emotional, married to a woman who is.

I turned to Irene. "So, Jack is learning to be more tolerant and not react to you. What would you say you're learning?"

"I'm working real hard to identify and express my feelings to him. But he always wants an explanation of *why* I feel upset. Sometimes you don't know why; you just know that you are."

Jack's response to Irene's distress took the familiar form of an obsessional person trying to comfort an emotional one: He barraged her with questions, all based on his own approach to emotion, which was to label and compartmentalize it.

Irene felt things strongly without always being able to put them into words. At these moments her husband could have comforted her by just being there, holding her perhaps, but certainly not demanding that she

---

[1] In writing this revision I noticed a Freudian slip here—he "needs" space, but she only "wants" closeness. Excuse me for a minute, my wife is trying to tell me something and I have to cover my ears and start humming.

stop crying and explain herself. The truth was that when Irene cried, Jack worried that it might be about him, so he felt accused. His comfort took the form of asking her to reassure him. "What's the matter?" really meant "Tell me you're not mad at me."

Jack went on to talk about Irene's anger as the reason he didn't listen better. When Irene approached Jack in an excitable way, he became anxious and responded by trying to be analytic or—if that failed—by distancing himself. His distance aggravated her emotionality, which then pushed him even further away. Their failure to listen to each other wasn't caused by Irene's emotionality or by Jack's anxiety; it was the combination.

Jack thought Irene could break the pattern by toning down her emotions. Irene thought Jack should learn to be a little more tolerant of her feelings. Even as they talked, they played out the familiar progression. Irene's rising pressure made Jack anxious and defensive—or, to look at the circular pattern from another angle—Jack's inability to accept what she was saying drove up her emotionality.

Finally I interrupted and told them the story of the North Wind. "One day the North Wind and the Sun were arguing about which was the most powerful force in nature. 'I can churn up the seas and drive a blizzard,' the North Wind said. 'Yes, but I can melt the snow and dry up a flood,' the Sun replied. Just then a man wearing a heavy overcoat happened by. 'I know how to settle this,' said the Sun. 'Let's see who can make that man take off his coat.' The North Wind blew hard. But the harder he blew, the more the man bundled up. Finally the Sun said, 'My turn.' The sun shone down its warmth, and the man unbuttoned his coat. The Sun shone warmer, and the man took off his coat."

Irene and Jack smiled broadly.

"Irene, sometimes you come on like the North Wind. And I don't blame you, because it's frustrating to feel shut out. And out of that frustration, either you give up or out comes the North Wind."

"You're right. I never thought of it that way."

At this point Jack, feeling relieved, opened up and started to talk about "needing" space.[2] He had a lot of pressure at work, and when he came home he needed time to decompress. And Irene was afraid to give

---

[2]See, I'm not the only one!

him the breathing room he needed, the freedom to read or go for a walk or spend time with his friends.

"Jack," I said, "I could tell you understood the difference between Irene being the North Wind and being the Sun. But you know, the guy wearing the coat is in the story too. It's both of them. The North Wind blows, and he bundles up, and so the North Wind blows more, and he bundles up more. He bundles up for a lot of good reasons—he has his moods, his job is stressful, he needs his space, he likes to read ... I respect those things. But the bundling up is part of the problem."

"I understand that," Jack said. He went on to say that he's been making an effort. But, he admitted, "It's not the easiest thing for me, to be close."

By now, the atmosphere in the session had changed. Jack and Irene had begun to see how they were locked into a pattern in which they both pushed each other to respond in a way they didn't like.

Once Irene learns to see very clearly that coming on strong only pushes Jack away, and *he* learns that keeping his distance only makes her more anxious and persistent, they can figure out how to break their halves of the cycle. Will that magically change everything? If you kiss a frog, will he turn into a prince? Maybe not right away.

Balancing Intimacy and Independence

In accommodating to each other, couples must negotiate the space between them as well as that separating their couplehood from the rest of the world.

When you become intimate with someone, physically and emotionally, you open up the boundary around your private self to let the other in close. Being in love is to want no distance between you, but a wall of privacy protecting the two of you from outside intrusion. This closeness and privacy make conversation intimate, with the obvious rewards and risks.

Minimal self-reliance exists between two people when they call each other at work all the time, when neither has separate friends or independent interests, if they come to view themselves only as a pair rather than also as two individuals. Under such pressure of togetherness conversation is constrained by the threat of conflict. If you're alone with someone on a lifeboat, you'd better not argue.

In contrast, people who put independence over connection do little together, have their own rooms, take separate vacations, have independent checking accounts, are more invested in their careers or outside relationships than in each other, and don't talk much. Listening is limited because they have so many distractions.

Most couples don't start out disengaged; the wall that grows up between them is a product of unresolved conflict. Often it's not specific transgressions so much as the not listening, the not hearing. They both feel as if the other doesn't care. That they do care very much but are too afraid of conflict to listen doesn't alter the feeling of being unappreciated. Some people pay a lot for peace.

Typically, partners come from families with differing degrees of separateness and togetherness. Each partner tends to be more comfortable with the kind of relationship he or she grew up with. Since these expectations differ, a struggle ensues over how much to share and how much to keep to yourself. This may be the most difficult aspect of learning to listen to a new mate—developing sensitivity to a different conversational style.

In the early stages of a couple's relationship, passion can mask difficulties in communicating. Some partners have broken away from their families, and they come together with an unchecked urgency for connection. Such fusion, such boundarylessness, the desideratum of love's young dream, is hard to sustain, especially when those in its thrall isolate themselves from family and friends. Couples who expect all their needs to be met in one all-fulfilling relationship are in for the rudest of awakenings. One reason people get too little out of intimate relationships is that they expect too much.

Tension in a couple can be resolved in one of three ways: working it out, triangulation, or distancing. When distancing between intimate partners is unchecked by a clear boundary around their relationship, the two often drift apart.

Brendan and Gina were very much in love when they married, also very young and unaware of how different their backgrounds were. Hers was a large, close-knit family whose watchword was togetherness. His was a small, fragmented family in which independence and personal achievement were the highest accomplishments.

In Brendan's opinion, Gina was addicted to attachment. She always wanted to talk. Even when they were watching TV or reading, she'd interrupt every few minutes to tell him something that popped into her head. It broke his concentration and made him furious. This he tried to signal indirectly by sighing or saying "Yes?" with a weary note in his voice. But Gina didn't seem to get the message.

Gina took closeness for granted and found Brendan's "coldness" and "detachment" selfish and mean. Why did he have to shut her out all the time?

They each had their own point of view, at best sporadically sympathetic to the other one. It's a sad and familiar story. Two young people with too great a disparity in their expectations to fit together easily, and too little experience to know how to work at it.

It wasn't really their differences that made the first few years together so painful; it was their inability to talk about them. Once a week or so, Gina would get fed up with Brendan's distance. At these times, Brendan was appalled by the meanness and exaggeration of her accusations. The worst was "You don't give a damn about anybody but yourself!" *How could she say such things?* He certainly couldn't listen. Feeling the frustration of not being heard, Gina would raise her voice, which only made Brendan shrink further into himself. Finally, Gina would break down in tears and sob, "Why are you so mean to me?" Brendan had the same question but only thought it, and never more than twice a day.

Like a lot of ill-matched couples, Brendan and Gina gradually did learn to live with each other. After a while they had children to cushion their couplehood. Gradually they learned to accommodate to each other. Gina got used to Brendan's silences and golfing with his friends. He learned to spend more time with her and the kids. But what they never learned very well was how to talk to each other. Brendan didn't talk to Gina because he thought she was unreasonable in her expectations and didn't respect his right to his own preferences. Gina continued to express her disappointment with Brendan's lack of involvement from time to time, but he never really did learn to listen. He listened well enough to pacify her—"I'm sorry"; "Yes, dear"—but not enough to understand how she felt. He wished she were different, he wished he could run away, and these thoughts kept him from ever really understanding or coming to terms with the real person he had married. Like a prisoner who thinks of nothing but escape, he never really did adjust to the realities of his relationship.

Pursuers and Distancers

Pursuers want more connection, which makes distancers feel pressured. The more she pursues, the more he distances; the more he distances, the more she pursues. It's a game without end, though it does have interruptions.

When pursuers get fed up with being rebuffed, they withdraw in hurt and anger. But after a while they start to get lonely, and then they begin the cycle all over again.

"Why Won't You Talk to Me?"

How can you convince a distancer that you are open and receptive to what he or she might be thinking and feeling? How can you convince a distancer of your openness without creating more pressure?

The person who withdraws doubts that anything good will come out of discussions. If you live with a distancer, you'll have to convince him or her that you're receptive to what he or she wants. Actually, you don't have to do that; you can just keep doing what you do, like most normal unhappily married people.

• • •

She wants to talk more. He wants to fight less.
To meet their own goals, both of them need to do more
of what the other one wants.

• • •

If you're a pursuer, try backing off. Focus less on the other person for a few days. This planned distance isn't the same as reactive distance—getting fed up and giving him the cold shoulder. Snubbing isn't the same as ignoring someone; it's an attempt to punish him with silence, which of course doesn't lessen your preoccupation with him. Instead of being passive-aggressive, increase your emotional investment in other things.

When you stop pursuing, notice what happens.[3] You'll probably find your anxiety rising. This is important. Consider how much of the pursuing is an attempt to cope with your own anxiety and lack of other avenues of satisfaction in your life.

Accept any forward movement on the part of a distancer—even if it's to complain. This is important. Pursuers say they want their partners to share feelings with them, but what they mean is positive feelings. A pursuer who experiments with shifting the pattern should avoid getting defensive about whatever the distancer does express. Distancers have feelings, too, but they keep them locked in tightly sealed compartments. If a distancer does start expressing feelings, try to listen without getting reactive.

If you're a distancer, pursuers are hard to live with. They put you on the defensive. It's hard to stop running when someone is chasing you. The first thing to realize is that it isn't just him or her chasing you; it's a pattern of pursuit and withdrawal. Instead of avoiding the pursuer, try initiating contact on your terms. Call your partner in the middle of the day; invite him or her to go for a walk. Say what's on your mind; ask what's on his or hers.

Change Is a Three-Step Process

If you shift your part in a pursuer–distancer pattern for a week, you'll discover that change is a three-step process: First you change. Second, your partner responds—usually in ways that are partly rewarding and partly annoying. Third comes your response to that response—either you change back, or you persist.

At what point do you usually give up? What could you do to persist in your effort to make changes in your relationship? Try sticking with a small change and notice what happens—how *you* feel—when the other person tries to get you to change back. Remember: it isn't what others do but how we react to what they do that tends to defeat us.

If a pursuer makes an effort to stop pursuing her partner, he may not immediately respond by moving toward her. The resulting distance might

---

[3]If you're a pursuer, you probably expected me to say something about your partner's behavior. Admit it!

make her feel cheated. She changed, but he didn't. At that critical juncture—the third step in the change process—she would either revert to her old style or persist, making an effort to remain calm, develop other interests, and give her partner space to discover his need for her.

Alternatively, if an emotional distancer decides to break the pattern by moving toward his partner, she might not immediately respond the way he wants her to. She might not, for example, be receptive to his opening up about things that are bothering him. She might be critical. If her response upsets him and he reverts to distancing, he might conclude, *I tried, but she'll never change.* But if he does change back, it wouldn't be because of how his partner responded; it would be because of how he responded to that response.

Another reason the pursuer–distancer dynamic isn't so easily resolved is that pursuers and distancers tend to have constitutionally different operating styles. Pursuers have an affinity for relationship time; distancers prefer time alone or activity together. (That's why some people are emotional distancers but sexual pursuers.) Pursuers tend to express their feelings; distancers avoid them. Pursuers have permeable boundaries and relate readily to a wide number of people. Distancers let down their defenses with only a select few.

Although each of us has a predominant operating style, the dynamics of complementarity trigger different roles in different relationships. A man may be a distancer with his mate and a pursuer with his mother. A woman may be a pursuer with her partner but a distancer from her stepfather.

Distancers are unsure of themselves in relationships; they depend on privacy for protection. Pursuing only makes them feel hounded.

• • •

To approach a distancer, don't push. Knock to enter. Give him time to anticipate company.

• • •

Distancers handle threatening issues by closing them off. Anxiety about these issues may not be acknowledged, but it is always present below the surface. The tension created by such unaddressed anxiety often triggers conflict in the relationship or emotional problems in one of the partners.

Emotional pursuers handle sensitive issues by talking about them over and over again in an anxious manner. The issues never become closed off,

and the emotionality surrounding them is never dealt with. For their partners, this repetitiousness is like salt poured on a wound.

Like most complementary patterns—overfunctioning/underfunction-
ing, strict/lenient, fast-paced/slow-paced—the pursuer–distancer dynamic
isn't static. Very little about relationships is static.

Accommodating Differences

Intimate partnership is a process in which two individuals restructure their
lives into a unit: The Couple. Friends invite The Couple over for dinner,
the IRS taxes The Couple, The Couple accumulates belongings. The two
separate personalities don't disappear, of course, but their relationship is
now a system, their fates interwoven.

The first priority of intimate partnership is mutual accommodation to
manage the details of everyday living. Each partner tries to organize the
relationship along familiar lines and pressures the other to accommodate.
They must agree on the big things, like where to live and whether and
when to have children. Less obvious, but equally important, they must
coordinate daily rituals, like what to watch on television, what to eat for
supper, when to go to bed, and what to do there. Unfortunately, there is a
thin line between accommodation and capitulation.

Lynn was just nineteen when her mother died. After the worst of
the grief gave way to emptiness, she decided to get out of New York and
move to Montana. When she got off the plane, she was stunned by the
intensity of the sunlight. The last of the snow was melting and the valley
blossomed. Summer came, stretched and yawned, and then it was early
fall. That's when the loneliness set in, and Lynn started wondering what
she was going to do with her life. Right about then she met Travis. After
all the boys she'd known in New York who couldn't stop talking about
themselves, Lynn took Travis's quietness for strength. She thought he was
the real deal. So when he asked her to share his trailer with him, it seemed
like the right thing to do.

A year later their relationship wasn't a lot better or a lot worse. Maybe
a wedding would do the trick. So Lynn gave Travis an ultimatum: either
they got married or she was moving out. But even walking down the aisle,

she found herself thinking *This is never going to last*. Afterward she got drunk, hoping to numb this giant step into the unknown.

Lynn got pregnant on the honeymoon, and two weeks later Travis joined the Air Force. When Travis was posted to Korea, he went ahead to get settled, and Lynn moved in with his parents. It was not a happy time. And so, six weeks later, when she boarded the plane for Inchon, it was with as much relief as anxiety.

When the jet lag wore off and reality settled in Lynn found herself alone all day with a baby in a tiny apartment. She'd written Travis to buy a car with an automatic transmission, because she couldn't drive a stick shift; but he hadn't listened. Not being able to drive sealed her isolation. When she tried to talk to Travis about it, he said, "You'll get the hang of it. Don't be such a baby." What could she say?

Unfortunately, Lynn neither insisted that Travis listen to how she was feeling nor asked how he was feeling. "I nagged," Lynn said. "I was angry and bitchy. Back then I wasn't very sure of what I was feeling, and so the frustration just built up and came out as attack. Instead of telling him how I was feeling, I'd say things like 'We never do anything; you never take me anywhere.' He always put it back on me. 'What's the matter with you?' That was his answer to all my complaints." She didn't really remember Travis's complaints; all she remembered was that he didn't listen to hers.

Going into the marriage, Lynn thought that if she did all the right things, Travis could become the man she wanted—loving and affectionate. She'd grown up with a self-absorbed father, and the question for her always had been *How do I make Daddy happy?* With Travis, she'd played the good wife, hoping for a payoff of affection and attention. But there was no affection; just sex. Lynn put up with not having her needs met because she wasn't sure how to put them into words.

When her frustration turned to bitterness, Lynn's conversations with Travis took on the form of combat. Each felt trapped and misunderstood, and both of them led with their defenses. After suffering so much neglect, Lynn was seized with rage when she tried to talk about her feelings. When she opened up on him with a mean mouth, his stomach knotted and he stopped listening. Once or twice, when she cornered him, he'd answer her accusations with an outburst of his own nursed resentment. Then they'd go back to avoiding each other.

The proximity forced on them in Korea may have kept them together longer than otherwise, or it may have put too much pressure on their shaky alliance. In any case, when Travis was posted back to the States and Lynn started school again, the marriage fell apart. With school and friends of her own, Lynn felt stronger and no longer willing to put up with a relationship that gave her so little satisfaction. Ironically, as Lynn started pulling away, Travis asked her to stay and, for the first time since the early days of the relationship, tried to listen to her. But it was too late.

Lynn said: "He wanted someone to mother him, to cook and clean and all that. I was willing to do it, and so he was happy. But when I wanted more from him, he couldn't deal with it, and he hated me. Then my independence gave him the room he needed, and so he started liking me again. But now I knew it had been a mistake to begin with." And so they ended it.

Travis and Lynn might have had an easier time adjusting to other mates. Maybe not. Second and third marriages don't fail because people keep picking the wrong partners; they fail because it's not differences that matter but how they're negotiated. Maybe Lynn did too much compromising. Maybe Travis did too little. He was a young man caught up in confirming his masculinity rather than achieving love, and perhaps he was afraid he'd lose himself by giving in. The trouble was, neither of them dared to listen to the other's point of view.

Travis and Lynn might have found a way to talk about their differences if they'd managed to be less emotionally reactive to each other. Instead of holding her feelings in until they exploded, Lynn might have approached Travis calmly (it isn't necessary to *feel* calm to *speak* calmly), saying, perhaps, "Something's bothering me and I need to talk to you. Is this a good time?"

●　●　●

The best way to tone down emotionality isn't to avoid talking about problems but to discuss them openly—before the upset boils over.

●　●　●

Travis thought that if he didn't listen to Lynn's complaints, he wouldn't have to deal with them—and he could avoid the anxiety her accusations made him feel. But he found out that feelings are like any other form of energy: if they don't find direct expression, they come out in other ways.

The way to reduce defensiveness is to stay calm and stay open. Don't interrupt, contradict, qualify, or change the subject. If you don't understand something, ask for clarification. Otherwise, shut up and listen.

"Why Can't a Woman Be More Like a Man?"

When the differences that attract turn out to be hard to live with, we may be tempted to think that a relationship might work best with a person as similar to us as possible. Actually, that's not true. With very similar partners there is the possibility for weaknesses to combine and create exaggerated, even destructive, imbalances. Two people with explosive tempers or who are both financially irresponsible often form disastrous unions.

Lynn told herself she married the wrong person. Travis was good-looking and smart, but he didn't know how to trust people with the truth about his feelings. A man dedicated to autonomy, married to a woman who prized togetherness. Travis, too, thought his mistake was choosing the wrong mate. He never suspected that the extravagant and desirable woman he fell in love with would turn out to be such a nag.

"I Heard You the First Time!"

Few complaints are more common from men than that the women in their lives nag. Whenever someone is perceived as nagging, it probably means she hasn't received a fair hearing for her concerns in a long time. When our feelings are listened to sympathetically, we experience a sense of understanding and release. If no one listens, we feel alone with our feelings.

"He never notices how much I do around here. I never get any help without having to beg for it."

Not being listened to makes people resentful. No wonder they come across as nagging.

"She acts like she's my mother. Doesn't she know I always get my share of the chores done?"

Lloyd *hates* Cathy's nagging.

Stop leaving the bedroom window open; don't turn the heat up any higher than sixty-eight degrees. Do this, do that. She's always bitching about something. This he says to himself, and he gets no argument.

Cathy hates that Lloyd never listens to her. "Why do I have to tell you the same things over and over again? Why can't you listen to a simple request?" This she says to him often. To her friend Samantha she complains, "I try to tell him something, and he just goes underground, with no warning—and I'm left there, all alone."

If You're Considered a Nag

In a series of conversations, each encounter bears the fruits and burdens of earlier ones. Persistent criticism creates a negative atmosphere and eventually results in the other person tuning the nagger out. It's like the Gary Larson cartoon in which a man is explaining something to his dog and all the dog hears is "blah-blah-blah."

The nagger becomes a nuisance. But what do you do if your repeated pleas to put dirty clothes in the hamper or clean up the mess in the bathroom go unheeded?

You're caught in the role of nag if, even though you know somebody isn't going to remember to do something, you keep bugging him anyway; you never ask for anything just once; you come at the other person in a critical or complaining way; you get annoyed by lots of things the other person does *and* you keep letting him know it; you appeal to what "should" be done rather than what you want; and the other person flinches when you make your request. You may not think of yourself as nagging, but if that's how the other person feels, he or she isn't likely to listen.

● ● ●

Nagging is in the ear of the beholder.

● ● ●

"Why Is Everything Always My Fault?"

Cut down on the number of things you ask people to do and the number of times you remind them. No fair, you say? You have a right to gripe? True, but asking less results in getting more.

Pick out your most important concerns, make your requests clearly, and make them sound like requests.

Listening is hard because it involves a loss of control, and if you're afraid of what you might hear, it may not feel safe to listen. Among the things that someone who feels nagged (even though he didn't listen the first twelve times) doesn't want to hear are blame and requests he doesn't think are open to discussion.

In all our communications we struggle to maintain our independence, to resist being controlled by others without sacrificing our involvement or losing their love. If someone hears your requests or complaints as implying power over him, he may resist—not because he's unwilling to do what you ask but because he's unwilling to accept the metamessage (implied or inferred) that you're the boss.

To avoid sounding overbearing, add "What do you think?" after making a request or a suggestion. This helps keep the airways open and the dialogue going. Emphasize how important the request is to you and be sure to understand the other person's perspective—"What do you think?" Then make sure that an agreement is really an agreement. If you aren't willing to accept "no," you can't trust "yes."

People other than our intimates are more likely to listen to us airing our frustrations because they know it isn't their fault. If you want to get heard more around the house, try telling your partner "I know it's not your fault," "I'm not blaming you." Then if he (or she) does listen, let him (or her) know you appreciate it. "I feel relieved that I can talk about this. Thanks for listening."

• • •

Saying "I really appreciate your listening to my feelings; it means a lot to me" encourages people to listen more.

• • •

Finally, if you want to get out of the role of a nag, try listening to the recalcitrant other's side of things. Maybe the husband who persists in running the washing machine with less than a full load feels that he has a right to do so if he wants. Perhaps the wife whose husband always has to remind her to buy beer when she gets groceries doesn't want to bring home beer—either because she wishes he would drink less or because she's resentful about something else.

Even if you don't agree with someone's reasons for not complying with your requests, he or she will feel a whole lot more like compromising if you listen to and acknowledge that point of view.

> ### Should You Say "No" More Often?
>
> Those who feel nagged are often people who have trouble saying "no." If a woman asks her husband to take out the garbage and it doesn't get done, probably there was a false sense of agreement to do it in the first place. Some people should say "no" more often.

How to Complain Without Starting a Fight

Directly related to nagging is complaining. The problem is that your expectations, often quite legitimate, that things should be different may provoke unwanted flare-ups if the other person feels attacked by what you say.

First decide whether what the other person does has a direct effect on you. Leaving dirty dishes around the house does, especially if you're the one who has to clean them up; your partner's ten extra pounds doesn't (unless you happen to own his or her body).

Consider your relationship to the person you're criticizing. It's one thing to tell your twelve-year-old that you want the lawn mowed more than twice a month. Saying the same thing to your husband (or wife) may make him react with *Who does she think she is, my mother?*

Partners who expect to be treated like adults may not take kindly to being told how to fold the laundry, load the dishwasher, or park the car. If you want these things done differently, maybe you should do them yourself.

If you decide you have a right to complain, consider whether or not the person is likely to change. Research has proven that, if properly motivated, some male *Homo sapiens* can learn to put dirty dishes in the sink. But few of us lose weight or start exercising just because someone else thinks we should.

If you've had to ask your partner a thousand times not to leave dirty dishes in the living room, maybe you should let it go. Maybe it's better to give up on some things—even if it's not fair—than to play the role of constant critic, a voice against which people learn to deafen themselves.

How to Complain

Do you have a tendency to hold your complaints in until you get fed up and then unload on the other person? Can you see how the consequences of such confrontations might reinforce your tendency to avoid complaining until you once again get good and mad?

How to complain? Start gently.

How you express criticism is important. Alert the person that you want to talk.

> "Something is bugging me, and I need to talk to you. How about tonight after work?"

> "I have a problem and I need to discuss it with you. Can we go for a walk after supper?"

Advance notice allows people to realize that something's coming and they'd better be prepared. Be sensitive to time and place. The best time to talk about difficult issues is when both of you are calm and relaxed. And alone.

That criticism is best given in private may seem obvious, but many people infuriate their partners by bringing up their faults in front of their friends or children. Another version of the same mistake is criticizing your partner's family or friends. It's okay for him to complain about his mother, but when you do you're crossing the line. Some people take advantage of being out with another couple to criticize their partners. Often they make a joke out of their comments. It isn't funny.

• • •

**If you have something to say to someone, tell them.
If you have something to say about someone's
friends or family, keep it to yourself.**

• • •

Telling someone "I have a problem" and "I need your help," even if your problem is about something he or she is doing, is more likely to be heard than direct criticism. Least likely to be heard is criticism framed as blame, put-downs, moralizing, or invidious comparisons.

"Why must you always ... ?"

"You never ... "

"You should ... "

"Why can't you be more like ... ?"

Emphasize your feelings, not the other person's shortcomings: "I wish you'd get dressed up when we go out. I feel more special when you wear your good clothes." This works better than, "Why do you always have to be so grungy?"

Describe how the situation is affecting you rather than being accusatory. Stick to behavior and make it clear that you're talking about what you like and don't like, not what's right or wrong. Focus on how the other person can help rather than on what he or she is doing wrong.

Even if you're the one with the complaint, remember to give the other person a turn. Mention your concern, but before elaborating, ask her how she feels about it. Don't get reactive if the other person gets defensive. Remember, you've just told her there's something wrong with what she's doing.

If you ask someone to make a change, and he agrees without saying much, he's less likely to follow through than if you inquire and acknowledge why he may not want to change or why changing might be hard for him.

Wendy told Hank that she needed more help chauffeuring the kids to their activities. He agreed. But Wendy went further and said, "I know you don't feel like it; otherwise you'd volunteer more often. When do you feel *least* like driving?"

Hank really appreciated this consideration of his feelings. (Feeling like it's okay to say no made it a lot easier to say yes.) He said he didn't mind taking the kids places on weekends or early in the evening, but he hated going out after nine on work nights. He also mentioned that it's easier for him if he knows a day in advance that he has to drive them somewhere.

Then Wendy went one step further and asked, "Anything else?"

Hank paused. Then he said, "Yes, there is. Frankly, I think you drive them far too many places. I don't think we should drive them wherever and whenever they want to go."

Wendy, who hadn't known Hank felt this way, said that the next time he disagreed he should say something. If she's willing to take them anyway, even if he isn't, she'll do the driving. "But," she added, "maybe you're right. Maybe I do drive them around too much."

On the way out of the movie theater, Ralph turned to Carmen and said, "Wow, that was a real stinker, wasn't it?" He went on to describe how a good story was ruined by Robin Williams's overacting and the director's sanctimonious moralizing.

Carmen didn't say anything. She had enjoyed the movie. She loved Robin Williams. Ralph's running the picture down was ruining it for her.

Since Carmen was the one who wanted to see this picture, she felt that Ralph was criticizing her taste and that while she was enjoying herself he'd been having a lousy time.

In fact, Ralph hadn't thought of this movie as Carmen's choice. She may have mentioned it first, but he had wanted to see it. And he hadn't had a lousy time. Far from it. He enjoyed laughing at parts of the movie, and he enjoyed laughing at some of its excesses.

What should you say on your way out of a movie you didn't like when you're with someone who apparently did? Nothing.

If two people both hate a movie or concert, their saying so brings them together. Shared experience, shared sensibilities. But if you enjoyed the performance, hearing someone else pick it apart spoils your fun.

Criticism of the movie or restaurant we liked feels like criticism of our taste. If you thought the food was lousy or the play was boring but sense that your companion liked it, let him savor his enjoyment. Save your criticism for later. Much later.

You Say Tom-ay-to, I Say Tom-ah-to

Your partner doesn't have the power to say what is and forever shall be or who's right and who's wrong. Even the person who puts things that way doesn't have the power to make it so; *you* give him that power if you react as though he did.

• • •

You don't have to agree in order to acknowledge that someone has a point.

• • •

The simple act of omission involved in not acknowledging what the other person is saying before countering with your own opinion may be the single greatest impediment to shared understanding. If we don't know that we've been heard, we're not about to hear what the other person is saying. Instead, we turn away or raise our voices. Maybe if we scream at her, she'll hear.

Emotional discussions should be kept as brief as possible. Don't unload everything. Doing so only makes the listener feel inundated, nailed to the wall, with just two choices: fight or flight.

Nowhere to turn. That's the way a lot of unhappy people feel about their relationships—trapped in the space of a relationship with someone who has some pretty stubborn ways. Accommodation means finding a way to fit together, but many people mistake fitting together as an all-or-nothing proposition.

Wise couples accept their differences and accommodate. But accommodating doesn't mean they must become two peas in a pod. Maybe she'll never be interested in politics. Maybe he'll never really get to like her parents. Rather than battle over these differences, or be untrue to themselves by giving in entirely, sensible partners avoid dwelling on subjects about which they don't agree. But instead of drifting apart or insulating themselves from each other, they search for alternative avenues of connection.

Adjusting to each other's realities requires tolerance and selective coming together. Mates may tire of hearing about each other's jobs, but they owe each other a few minutes of listening at the end of the day. (Asking questions may make familiar stories more interesting.) But couples must also figure out which subjects are most rewarding to talk about together. The same balance applies to activities other than talking.

When Dennis returned from playing golf on Sunday morning, Lorraine was still in bed, so he took off his clothes and crawled in beside her.

When he kissed her awake, she gave him a dubious look. It wasn't what he'd hoped for, but over the years he'd learned the difference between a red light and a yellow one. When they were first married, Dennis expected Lorraine to be ready for sex on demand. When she tried to slow him down and later said no, he felt rejected and avoided her altogether. Now he read her look as saying that she was happy to see him but not really in the mood to make love. They did a lot of talking with their eyes, but he made himself say, "Let's just hug a little." They did, and after a while Lorraine relaxed enough to become more affectionate. In the end they did make gentle love.

After lunch Dennis mentioned that he was going to watch football for a while. Once he'd expected to watch football all day on Sunday, and Lorraine, who came from a family that didn't follow the national obsession, would get very angry. For years they'd alternate between his watching and her fuming and his not watching and feeling resentful. This day he watched the first half while she had a long phone conversation with a friend, read the paper, and occasionally looked up when the crowd roared. At halftime she asked if he wanted to go to the movies. He did. Movies were one thing they never had to compromise about. They went to see *Oceans Twenty-Seven* but didn't go shopping afterward, as he knew she would have liked and she knew he would not have. After supper, they watched television for a while, until Lorraine went into the other room and read. It was a nice day.

As this example illustrates, listening, in its full sense, means taking each other into account. Dennis listened to Lorraine signaling her mood; later she listened to his wish to watch football, and between them they found a balance between separateness and togetherness.

In spite of the large emotions involved, marriage isn't about monumental issues; it's about little things, about everydayness, about knowing that tomorrow morning you'll wake up with a new chance to work at it, to get it a bit more wrong or right.

Getting Beyond Bitterness

Although couples who survive the break-in period tend to mellow, they still go through cycles of closeness and distance. Some conflicts are resolved, others are avoided, and some keep cropping up from time to time. Arguments still occur, but the nature of these quarrels should change over time. They become less bitter and less violent. There is less blaming and a greater feeling that both of you are in the same boat. If arguments don't become less frequent, less intense, and shorter, partners would do well to see what they're doing to keep resentment present and listening absent.

Successful couples learn that attempting to induce unilateral change using emotional manipulation—complaining, cajoling, sweet-talking, nagging, guilt-tripping, getting angry—doesn't work very well. When empathy doesn't come easy, successful partners work at it—making themselves listen even when it's hard. (You don't have to *feel* sympathetic to listen. Sometimes showing concern works from the outside in, the way smiling can put you in a good mood.)

Problems arise when partners keep too many secrets, say yes when they don't mean it, or withhold the truth of their feelings because they're afraid of arguments. The broken promises that result from being afraid to say no are too great a price to pay for avoiding honest argument. Learning to say no enables you to say yes and mean it. If you're wishing that your partner would realize this, ask yourself, why would someone lie to you?

Trust allows people to relax into themselves. Being honest is central to establishing this trust, as is being open, listening to and acknowledging the hard things your partner says. Love that grows out of self-respect is love for ourselves as we are, not for a partial and carefully selected portion. The person who hesitates to speak wonders if it's safe to broach certain subjects. The person who never opens up to you has already decided.

• • •

If you want the truth from someone, you must make it safe for him or her to tell it.

• • •

Unfortunately, even with the best of intentions, some couples reach a point where they get bogged down in bitterness. Pursuers get sick of pursuing and distancers get tired of the pressure, until one or both of them pulls back to what family therapist Phil Guerin calls an "island of invulnerability."[4] Anger builds to resentment, and two people who once thrilled to each other now give up on each other. Retreating to an island of

---

[4]Philip Guerin, Leo Fay, Susan Burden, and Judith Kautto, *The Evaluation and Treatment of Marital Conflict* (New York: Basic Books, 1987).

invulnerability is cold comfort. But even loneliness sometimes feels better than constant conflict.

Mates bogged down in bitterness can take a step toward releasing themselves from frozen hopes by taking a hard look at those hopes. If you're willing to let go of blaming and look for a way back together, examine your expectations. Are your conflicts based on a desire for a partner who is fundamentally different from the one you married? If you're irritated with your partner for being who he or she is, rather than about some particular behavior, then you are in the wrong relationship. The only things worth fighting about are the things that can be changed.

People come to intimate partnership with a self-contradictory pair of expectations. They expect their partners to duplicate the good aspects of their own families and make up for the bad. To make matters worse, these expectations are often directed at a partner's limitations rather than his or her strengths. ("I know he could be a more sociable person, if he only tried.")

Don't judge your partner by measuring him (or her) against your strengths; measure him by his strengths. We all want to be appreciated for who we are.

• • •

No one benefits when weaknesses or shortcomings become the principal focus of attention in a relationship.

• • •

To move away from bitterness, concentrate on your partner's virtues. See if some of the things you find objectionable are actually the downside of attributes you appreciate, that may have attracted you in the first place. If your partner were different in ways you'd like, he or she would also be different in ways you wouldn't like. Request changes of certain behavior, but don't punish your partner for what you consider misbehavior. Find your way to acceptance. Tenderness will follow.

With maturity, the human quest moves from the outside in, from conquering the world to struggling with ourselves—to be who we are and to be connected to others. Looking for love that will simultaneously recreate and undo the past, we latch on to someone and hope for the best.

New couples are ripe with possibility. Over time they become structured into a system, organized by the demands of living together and perhaps raising a family. As we've seen, the process that transforms two people into a pair is based on accommodation and boundary making.

At first, patterns of behavior in a couple are free to vary; later they become entrenched. But even then, change is possible. The key is complementarity. Those who would remake their own luck must learn to see the annoying things their partners do as one part of a pattern, a pattern that connects two people together in cycles of action and reaction. Look to your part.

*   *   *

What I've tried to show in this chapter is how a better understanding of the joys and sorrows of intimate partnership comes from looking beyond personalities to the patterns of interaction between them. Problems, it turns out, are more likely to be resolved, not by trying to change what your partner does, but by changing how you respond to it. Once you discover that the more you do X, the more he does Y—or he realizes that the more he does Y, the more you do X—either one of you can change the pattern by altering your own input. But when a twosome becomes a threesome, things get a little more complicated.

As I'll explain in the next chapter, to understand what goes on in families, it's necessary to look beyond the dynamics of interaction between two people to the overall organization of the whole group. I hope these considerations will prove useful to you in understanding what goes on between you and every other member of your family.

Exercises

1. Identify three negative assumptions about your partner. During the next week look for evidence contrary to any of those negative assumptions. (Hint: Consider motivation, not just behavior.)

2. Look back over the last few days and try to list three or four times when your partner did something good for the relationship and you failed to let him or her know that you appreciated it.

3. In your relationship, are you more of a pursuer or a distancer? Why do you do that? Are you afraid of change? Afraid of conflict? What are you seeking when you pursue? Are you looking for mutual benefit or for changes that would mainly benefit you? What do you distance yourself from? Why does what you're avoiding make you anxious? What would you gain by shifting from avoidance to approach once in a while?

If your partner is a distancer, what do you think he or she is avoiding? What can you do to reassure your partner that what he or she is afraid of isn't going to happen?

If your partner is a pursuer, what does he or she want from you? How can you initiate giving more of what he or she wants in a way that doesn't make you feel like a victim?

4. A friend is someone with whom you can relax and be yourself. You can ask a friend for a favor. A friend is someone you can count on. A friend is someone you can talk to. For women this kind of talking tends to occur face to face, whereas for men, talking with friends tends to occur while they are doing something.

What would happen if you went out of your way to be a friend to your partner for a few days? Why don't you try it and see?

5. Make a list of your differences from your partner that he or she has trouble accepting. For each one, how would it affect your relationship if he or she were to become more accepting?

Make a list of your partner's differences that you have trouble accepting. For each one, how would it affect your relationship if you made an effort to become more accepting?

11

• • •

"Nobody around Here
Ever Listens to Me!"

How to Listen and Be Heard
within the Family

As we've seen, the quality of understanding between people isn't fixed in character but depends on the *process* of their interaction. The advantage of seeing the process of relationships is flexibility. What can be recognized as a pattern of mutual influence can be changed. But there's a catch. Once children arrive on the scene, the dynamics of couplehood are no longer sufficient to explain what goes on in the family. Now, it isn't just how two people interact that can lead to problems in understanding but how the overall organization of the family affects every single individual and combination of family members. Patterns of communication in families are hard to change because they're embedded in powerful but unseen structures.

Family Structure

Families, like other groups, have rich possibilities for satisfaction. (Don't we marry and bring children into the world with clear and simple hopes for happiness?) Walt Whitman said, "I contain multitudes." The same could be said of family relationships, though, sadly, many congeal into limited and limiting molds.

• • •

Listening is an art that requires openness to each other's uniqueness and tolerance of differences.

• • •

As they are repeated, family transactions foster expectations that establish enduring patterns.[1] Once these patterns are established, family members use only a fraction of the full range of behavior available to them. The first time the baby cries or the in-laws come to visit, it's not certain who will do what. Will the load be shared? Will there be a quarrel? Will one person get stuck with all the work? Soon patterns are set, roles assigned, and things take on a sameness and predictability.

When a mother tells her son to put away his toys and he ignores her until his father yells at him, an interactional pattern is initiated. If it's repeated, it creates a structure in which the father becomes the disciplinarian and the mother is the permissive parent.

• • •

Family members tend to have reciprocal and complementary functions; the more one parent does for the children, the less the other is likely to do. Where one partner is weak, the other is strong.

• • •

The Possibilities in Every Pair

A family system differentiates and carries out its functions through *subsystems*. Every individual is a subsystem, and dyads (such as husband–wife or mother–child), as well as larger groups, make up other subsystems, determined by generation, gender, and function.

Individuals, subsystems, and whole families are demarcated by interpersonal *boundaries*, emotional barriers that regulate the amount of contact with others. Boundaries protect the autonomy of the family and its

---

[1]Salvador Minuchin and Michael P. Nichols, *Family Healing* (New York: The Free Press, 1993).

subsystems. A rule forbidding phone calls at dinnertime establishes a boundary that insulates the family from outside intrusion. When children are permitted to freely interrupt their parents' conversations, the boundary separating the adults from the children is blurred.

Subsystems inadequately shielded by boundaries limit the potential of these subgroups. If parents always step in to settle their arguments, children won't learn to fight their own battles. Similarly, when in-laws are too actively involved in a couple's affairs, the couple will be slow to develop their own resources.

These days when work and after-school activities consume so much of our lives, we have limited time for ourselves and less time for our families. In the few hours we do have with our families, many of us are reluctant to exclude some members of the family so that others can do things together—such as a father taking a daughter to a basketball game or a mother and son taking in a movie together. This is unfortunate.

• • •

Time alone together allows every pair in the family a chance to talk and freedom to listen.

• • •

The most obvious example of a relationship that suffers without time alone together is the one between wife and husband.

Lewis felt that he'd lost his wife to the children. Once Iris had been his friend and lover as well as his wife. Deciding to have kids and the pregnancy and the birth and those first few wonderful, exhausting months of babyhood brought them closer together. Then, as Lewis saw it, Iris pulled motherhood over her head like a blanket. They were still friends, sort of, but they were more parents than anything else. They rarely listened to each other because they rarely talked. When Lewis decided to move beyond cursing fate and casting blame, he found that the simple act of spending time alone together with Iris was the first step in revitalizing their marriage. (In the process he discovered that two people who aren't spending time together aren't just busy; they're also dissatisfied with the listening they're getting.)

Parents need time alone with each of their children. One of the best ways for parents to listen to their children is to arrange little outings with each one. Once a week isn't too much to aim for. Even if a child has a good relationship with a parent, conversation and intimacy are easier away from everyday distractions. The time a parent spends taking a child out to dinner or for a hike or on a bus ride into the city may well be the best time in both of their lives. Every pair has its possibilities.

Now let's look at how some familiar structural flaws create problems in listening.

When Boundaries Are Blurred

The two biggest mistakes parents make in listening to their children both involve blurred boundaries: failing to establish control over their children's behavior and interfering too much in their lives.

The most important thing to keep in mind when listening to children is the difference between allowing them to *say* what they want and letting them *do* what they want. When a child says "I don't want to go to bed," he or she is expressing a feeling and making a request. A wise parent distinguishes between the two and acknowledges the feeling before ruling on the request.

Of course children don't want to go to bed! They might miss something. Staying awake is their way of clutching at life. Parents who blur the distinction between expression and action get into foolish debates with their children. They say "I don't care what you want; you're going to bed anyway." Or they try to convince children that they're tired, as though obeying the rules depended on agreeing with them.

Parents who confuse love with leniency often fail to enforce their rules. Mistaking permissiveness for understanding and democracy for respect, such parents confuse their children about who's in charge and end up too anxious about controlling the children's behavior to be able to listen to their feelings. The dichotomy between authority and understanding is a false one; actually, they go hand in hand.

The most common alternative to effective discipline is nagging. Constant bickering with children wounds their pride and does more to engender insecurity than to establish parental authority. Effective parents take control early in their children's lives and use it sparingly.

• • •

Children learn from the consequences of their behavior.
If the consequence of every third or fourth thing they do

is that their parents nag them, children learn that their parents are nags and that they are a nuisance.

• • •

The boundary that makes it easier for parents to listen to their children because they are in charge is related to one of the crucial elements in listening: acknowledging what the other person says before responding with what you have to say.

Remember Tommy, the boy whose father lectured him on the evils of anger? If only his father had first acknowledged what Tommy was feeling, the boy might have been more open to his father's message. Seeing Tommy storm upstairs and slam his door, his father might have said, "It's frustrating when the mower doesn't work, isn't it?" or "Sounds like you had a bad time."

Being a parent in charge doesn't make you a good listener, but it does release you from some of the anxiety about control that gets in the way of listening.

Suppose a little girl runs into the kitchen saying, "Look, I caught a caterpillar!" The mother who responds with "Go wash your dirty hands!" is obviously deflating the child's enthusiasm. Saying, "Yes, that's nice, but go and wash your hands" isn't very responsive either.

• • •

"Yes, but … " is never enough. The *but* drowns out the *yes*.

• • •

"Yes, but … " isn't a real acknowledgment. Like adults, children need to feel heard before they're open to a new thought. If a mother were to take a minute to acknowledge her child's enthusiasm, she might say, "What a pretty caterpillar," or "Hey, wow! Good for you!" The little girl, feeling heard and appreciated, might then wash her hands without needing to be told, especially if she knows that's the rule.

• • •

If children suffer when the boundary between them and their parents is too diffuse, so do the parents. Parents too actively involved in their children's lives tend to be less actively involved with each other. This may not be obvious to some parents because

they do so many things together. But how many
things do they do together without the children?

* * *

Emotional Triangles

When he came downstairs, Marshall was surprised to see his teenage
daughter sitting at the breakfast table sipping hot chocolate. Before he
could ask why she was still home, Paula jumped up and threw her arms
around his neck: "No school!" Looking out the window, Marshall saw the
yard blanketed in white.

Assuming the driving would be bad, Marshall decided to wait until
after nine before going to work. By that time the roads would be clear and
the worst of the traffic would be gone. While he boiled water and ground
the beans for coffee, Paula built a fire in the fireplace. When the coffee was
ready and the fire blazing, they sat on the couch to watch the flames and
share something that had lately gone out of their relationship: time alone
together.

Just then the front door flew open, and in walked Paula's boyfriend.
"Guess what? School's canceled!"

"Hi, Jerry," Marshall said, none too enthusiastically. Then he went
upstairs to his study. He didn't exactly slam the door, but he didn't close it
very gently either.

Paula and her father, who had been so close, were growing further and
farther apart in this, her last year of high school. As Marshall sat there brooding about how Paula seemed to drop everything, including her homework,
when Jerry was around, he knew he was wrong. Daughters grew up and had
boyfriends; a father had to accept these things. He knew he was wrong to be
so resentful of Jerry, and now he had that bitterness as well to swallow.

When Paula was born, Marshall vowed never to be one of those
fathers who said, "I'll play with you tomorrow." What a remarkable thing it
was to be a daddy, gifted and burdened with the power to bestow moments
of total joy. As Paula grew older, they still did special things together, but
he noticed that her pleasure in his company was no longer entirely sponta-
neous; he knew that at least part of the time they spent together now was
only to please him.

Two weeks later Jerry broke up with Paula. She cried but showed no sign of real grief. These things happen. Marshall couldn't help being secretly relieved and said so to Elaine.

On Monday Paula said she couldn't face going to school. Couldn't she stay home, just for one day? It seemed little enough to ask. That afternoon Elaine decided to come home early and cheer Paula up with a little shopping expedition. Finding Paula asleep in her room, still in her nightgown, was no great surprise. After all, it wasn't easy being seventeen and having your heart broken. Elaine never knew what made her go into the hall bathroom, where she found the empty bottle of aspirin in the wastebasket.

Paula spent four weeks at Twin Oaks on the adolescent unit, where she learned the importance of giving voice to her feelings. When she discovered her anger, she started raging at her mother for always wanting everything to be "nice" and for thinking that shopping could be the answer to her problems. Her mother then did a surprising thing: she listened. But when Paula directed her anger at Marshall, telling him that he'd been unfair to blame her for growing up and having a boyfriend, Marshall got defensive. Nothing hurts like the truth.

During the last week of Paula's stay in the hospital, Jerry came to visit her, and after she was discharged, they started seeing each other again. Marshall was not happy.

Aside from his earlier objections about Jerry, he didn't think it was a good idea for Paula to put herself back into a vulnerable position so soon. His mind filled with bitter thoughts—about this callow boy who'd hurt his daughter, and might do so again, and about Paula's unforgiving anger at *him*. Well, maybe bitter thoughts were easier than wondering how a father lets go of his daughter.

Now when Jerry came around, Marshall was barely civil. He wanted to talk to Paula about not becoming dependent, about the importance of having many friends, but he was afraid of her anger, and his own. So he started complaining to Elaine.

Paula, too, complained to her mother. "Why is Daddy so unfair?"

Time passed, and the crisis—that's what Marshall called it; he couldn't bring himself to say "suicide attempt"—began to seem unreal and long ago. Routine reasserted itself, and the only truly tense moments were occasions on which Paula wanted to go somewhere with Jerry and Marshall looked grim and said nothing. If Paula pressed him, he said sarcastically, "Ask your mother." He felt angry and bereft, but increasingly less so.

Winter passed, and then it was spring. After graduation Paula broke off with Jerry, saying she wanted to have her last summer at home free to be with her friends. Men, she had learned, can be pretty possessive.

In D. H. Lawrence's *Sons and Lovers*, Paul Morel, the young artist, doesn't feel free to become his own person until his adored mother releases him from her jealous love by dying. In the last scene, when Paul's sweetheart, Miriam, asks if he is now free to marry, he says no. He's become free to go his own way.

One of the great themes of literature is the oedipal conflict—a child's passionate attachment to one parent and rivalry with the other. In real families, children fall in and out of love with both parents many times. We expect fathers to become antagonistic to their sons—and hope they will grow out of it. But when a father becomes alienated from his daughter, as Marshall did, we seek explanations in character and circumstance. Maybe Marshall was too attached to his daughter to tolerate a rival. Maybe he was too stubborn to let go. Or perhaps we can be more generous and say that it was only natural for him to worry about Paula's relationship with Jerry, considering what happened.

The trouble with these explanations is that they may account for the conflict but not why it wasn't resolved. Most family conflicts eventually get worked out—*if* the individuals involved are willing to listen to each other.

The Cotherapist in Family Therapy

Families, as you may have noticed, sometimes get stuck in ruts. Their problems are reinforced by the interlocking actions of more than one person. That's why the first family therapists described families as homeostatic systems that resist therapeutic efforts to change them. Over many years of practice, I learned to look in every family for a cotherapist—one person willing to set aside blaming and take the first step toward transforming family patterns by changing his or her own contribution. It takes more than one person to make a family what it is, but one person can initiate change. Could you be that person in your family?

When Paula felt the innocent indignation of being misunderstood by her father, it seemed only natural to turn to her mother. Likewise, when Marshall worried about Paula's seeing Jerry again, it seemed reasonable to complain to his wife. In turning away from each other and detouring their dispute through Elaine, Paula and her father created a triangle, one of the great roadblocks to listening.

Take a minute to think about your most difficult relationship in your family. Chances are you thought of your spouse, or maybe one of your parents, or a child, or perhaps one of your in-laws. Actually, the relationship you thought of is almost certainly between you and that person and one or more other parties.

• • •

Virtually all emotionally significant relationships between two people are shadowed by a third— a relative, a friend, even a memory.

• • •

The most notorious triangle is the extramarital affair. An affair might compensate for something missing in a marriage, but as long as one's emotional energy is invested elsewhere, there's little chance of improving the primary relationship. Similarly, if a young husband or wife remains overly attached to his or her parents and runs to them with complaints about the spouse, the couple in formation may never work out their difficulties. Some triangles seem so innocent that we hardly notice their destructive effect. Many parents can't seem to resist complaining once in a while to their children about their mates. "Your mother's *always* late!" "Your father *never* lets anyone else drive." These interchanges seem harmless enough. If you're really upset about something, you need to talk about it, right?

• • •

When you hear a story in which one person is a victim and the other is a villain, you're being invited into a triangle.

• • •

If something's really bothering you and you're afraid to talk about it— afraid you won't be listened to—the urge to confide in someone is almost overwhelming. The trouble with triangles isn't that seeking sympathy is wrong. The problem is that triangles can become chronic diversions that corrupt and undermine listening in family relationships.

Mary was a twenty-year-old, single mother who came to the clinic because she was having trouble controlling her three-year-old. After I'd listened to her for about forty minutes, Mary confessed that she'd been hitting the baby and was afraid she might hurt her. I was alarmed, so I asked Mary to bring Tamara to the next session.

Mary, who lived alone and had few friends, related to her little daughter like a playmate. When the baby was building a tower with blocks, Mary grabbed away some of the blocks to make her own tower, insisting that the baby "share." Later in the session, when I was trying to talk with Mary about her life as a single mom and Tamara started throwing blocks, Mary yelled at her—"Quiet down, okay? I'm talking to the doctor"—but didn't follow up. Tamara looked up for a minute and then continued throwing blocks. She was used to ignoring her mother.

Over the next two sessions I helped Mary understand what it means to be a mother-in-charge. Parents take charge by being parental, which consists of two things: nurture and control. (The latter makes the former easier.) Mary learned not to try to control everything the baby did but that when she did need to enforce a rule to do so with a clear, direct message and then follow through with consequences. Becoming more confident of her authority made it easier for her to be more tolerant of Tamara. The language of small children is a language of action; "listening" to them means letting them take the lead in play.

Mary was a quick learner, and her relationship with Tamara improved rapidly. They started getting along better; but in the fifth session, Mary reported that she was still having trouble with Tamara at home. It was only then that she told me that often when Tamara was punished, she'd run down the hall to her grandmother's apartment. Instead of supporting her daughter's authority, Mary's mother tried to comfort Tamara by telling her not to worry, "Grandma loves you."

The grandmother's interference with her daughter's discipline may strike you as too obviously misguided to be of much relevance to the problems of listening in your own life. But aren't you playing the same game whenever you take one person's side against another?

Most family problems are triangular. That's why working with two people may have limited results. Teaching a mother techniques for disciplining her son won't resolve the problem that she's overinvolved with the boy as a result of her husband's emotional distance. Similarly, working on a couple's communication may not bring them closer together as long as their number-one priority is children or their careers.

Are triangles always a problem? No. Sometimes you just *have to* talk to someone else. For example, when I complain to my friends about my wife nagging me to take out the garbage, it's because my wife doesn't understand that I don't always feel like doing it. Besides, if I tried to discuss this directly with her, we might get into tedious and unnecessary issues, like fairness and inequality and so on.

When Rigid Boundaries Keep People Apart

Some people establish rigid boundaries, so restrictive that they permit too little contact, resulting in *disengagement*. Disengaged people are independent but isolated. On the positive side, this fosters autonomy. If parents don't hover over their children, telling them what to do and refereeing their battles, the children will be forced to develop their own resources. On the other hand, disengagement limits affection and nurture.

Being listened to by their parents is how children build confidence in their powers of communication. Parents may not always listen, but for a day care worker in charge of eight toddlers at once, it's almost impossible to listen more than very briefly.

A visit to your child's school might result in the sober realization of how little children are listened to and might inspire you to reoccupy center stage in your children's school-dominated lives. Spending time with your children—without turning everything into a struggle for control—helps displace peer pressure and pedagogy that compel your children to conform or rebel, both of which undermine their efforts to discover themselves.

● ● ●

The way to help children figure out who they are is to listen to them.

● ● ●

Disengagement is a behavioral description for lack of involvement—spending time together, sharing activities, talking. People who are disengaged aren't necessarily uncaring, even if they do seem to spend a lot of time pursuing their own interests. Often these individuals are using distance and displacement to insulate their own sensitivities.

Suzanne and Rick were worried about their son's difficulty making friends. The boy's lack of friends, as it turned out, was nothing serious, little more than a ticket of admission to therapy. Actually, Suzanne was more concerned about the lack of closeness between her and Rick. She complained of his distance and of his not thinking about her needs, but she talked in an anxious, unclear way, circling her feelings, never really saying flat out what she meant.

Rick tried to listen but wasn't very good at it. Perhaps he recoiled at the underlying whininess of Suzanne's complaints. Suzanne also mentioned—"by the way"—that she was seeing an individual therapist. When I asked why, she said she needed someone to understand how she felt. (*Oh, great*, I thought. *She's using a therapist as her confidant at the same time she's trying to create a more confiding relationship with her husband.*)

The hard core of Suzanne's and Rick's problem with intimacy wasn't just that they were busy or that the wild happiness they once knew had faded or simply that they'd gotten out of the habit of being close. It was that they had trouble talking and listening to each other. Her contribution was holding back her complaints and then venting them in emotional outbursts. His contribution was not listening hard enough to penetrate Suzanne's complaints and hear her loneliness and not speaking up about his own grievances. He made a typical unconscious bargain: if he wasn't satisfying her demands, he'd better not make any of his own.

After a while they started getting through to each other. Suzanne was able to be more direct with her requests when she realized how she'd learned to avoid asking for what she wanted by observing her mother's constant complaining. Rick worked harder at listening and harder at speaking up. Then Suzanne made what felt like a confession. For years she'd spent hours every day confiding in her journal. She spoke of it almost like a child's invisible friend. This, then, was Rick's rival.

Is it wrong to complain about your spouse to an individual therapist? Is it wrong to keep a diary? Of course not. But the more you confide your feelings to someone or something other than the people you want to get closer to, the less pressure you feel to improve those relationships.

Disengaged relationships don't exist in a vacuum. To close the distance between you and someone you love, keep two things in mind: You catch more flies with honey than with vinegar. And if you want to close the distance in a disengaged relationship, be prepared to hear some complaints. Disengagement isn't just distance; it's protective distance.

When Closeness Smothers Intimacy

Sometimes the boundary separating family members from the rest of the world is so rigid that relationships become enmeshed, offering closeness at the expense of autonomy. Isolation—from conversation, broadly speaking, with the rest of the world—puts too much pressure on any relationship. Intimacy grows with time together and time apart.

Some people are togetherness oriented. They value closeness and connection, but these values can actually reduce intimacy if they result in pressure to conform. To achieve genuine closeness, you must respect every family member's sovereign individual experience, their right to their own feelings and their own point of view.

Enmeshed relationships can comfort like a warm coat on a cold day or chafe like a wool blanket on a hot night. Children enmeshed with their parents become dependent. They're less comfortable by themselves and may have trouble relating to people outside the family.

We usually assume that parental involvement with children is a good thing: if children are having problems, their parents must not be sufficiently engaged. In some cases this is true. But sometimes the problem is parental overinvolvement, robbing children of room to be themselves—to have problems, make mistakes, and learn to chart their own course.

A clear boundary between the generations puts parents in charge, allows them to claim their own rights and privacy, and helps them respect the children's autonomy within their own orbit.

When family therapists encounter mothers enmeshed with their children, they certainly don't blame mothers for this arrangement (as though a family's structure were the unilateral doing of one of its members). Oh, no, they would never do that!

Enmeshment, unfortunately, *is* usually blamed on mothers. Who else? They're the ones smothering their children, aren't they?[2] Blaming mothers for a family structure that leaves them neglected by their husbands and overinvolved with their children is like saying that a car without spark plugs won't go because the pistons don't fire. Even infants and mothers engulfed in the blissful intimacy of baby love need paternal involvement. They need a supporter and a confidant, not a frustrated competitor.

• • •

Children need attachment? So do their parents.

• • •

Some of the overidentification of mothers with their children may be due to their being wedded to their roles as selfless servants. Critics often suggest that enmeshed mothers should have more of a life of their own. Meaning careers, doing things, spending time with friends, and so on. But some of what they need is the experience of being listened to and empathized with. It's getting the listening you need that makes you strong, not trying to go it alone.

Parents need to be united. But most parents have different opinions on at least some issues involving their children. What should they do? They should talk about their opinions and listen to each other. Then they can decide how to act.

Forming a United Front

To forge an alliance that works, both parents must yield on some issues to gain in unity. *Accommodation* is the process by which people adjust their differences to come together. It is the mechanism of compromise, sometimes a deliberate result of negotiation, sometimes the result of instinctive adjustments. Unified family leadership is based on communication and compromise between parents and then presented to the children as one policy. Most parents eventually discover how important it is to accommodate their differences in order to present a united front. Similarly, as many people eventually discover, it's learning to accept each other, not trying to improve your partner, that makes couples last.

---

[2]Most people still harbor ancient grudges against the hand that rocked the cradle.

• • •

**When children continue to misbehave, you can bet
that one parent isn't backing the other up.**

• • •

If you don't feel supported by your partner in parenting, if you get stuck with all the driving or always have to be the one to enforce the rules, don't put all the blame on your partner. Maybe he or she disagrees with what you're doing. Try asking.

"I get the feeling you don't really agree with my way of handling this. Maybe you don't think I'm interested in your opinion—but I am. I'd really like to hear what you think."

Parenting is also an excellent place to observe the other side of complementarity—polarization. Instead of coming together on certain issues, parents push each other further apart. If one is too strict, the other may become too lenient. The more one harps at the children, the more the other tries to compensate by being indulgent.

Polarization is what happens when the controls on your electric blanket get switched. The first attempt by either of you to make it warmer or colder will set off a cycle of mutual maladjustment.

Small differences can drive couples to antagonistic opposites. A mother whose threshold for telling the kids to quiet down is only slightly higher than her husband's may never get the chance to discipline them if he always shushes them before she feels the need. Every time he reprimands the kids, she'll feel he's being too harsh. If she complains about his impatience, he'll get angry. Family life then becomes a battleground, where instead of sticking together, two parents become adversaries in a game where everybody loses.

Why do couples accommodate on some issues and polarize on others? Because we compromise where we're able but polarize in response to our own inner conflicts.

The engine that drives conflicts within us to become conflicts between us is projection. This dynamic comes into play when an ambivalent balance between pairs of conflicting impulses (dependence–independence, emotional expression–restraint, desire–anxiety, privacy–companionship) is resolved by projecting one's own motivation onto the other person. A man (or woman) who's afraid of anger may express it through passive control that provokes his (or her) partner. When they fight, she gets angry and he gets hurt. The man who feels only hurt may be seething with rage but remains unaware of those feelings as long as he has an obliging mate to act out his anger for him. In the process, the partner who shows anger may be able to avoid facing inner feelings of helplessness.

• • •

**Polarized mates fight in each other what
they can't accept in themselves.**

• • •

Projection and polarization turn couples into antagonists and prevent partners from integrating latent possibilities in the self—because these are played out by the other. The tough man may be unable to integrate his softer side to the extent that his wife acts emotional and helpless. His dependent wishes and vulnerability are repudiated because they're seen as her domain. She then becomes a dependent and demanding wife. This is one reason men take revenge for their dependency—that bottomless need for mother-love—by bullying and belittling their wives for exhibiting the needs they themselves don't dare express.

In our day, gender differences have permeated public consciousness. No longer do we believe that men are strong and women weak. Yet what is the current vogue of celebrating women's uniqueness if not stereotyping updated? It's hard for husbands and wives to work at partnership when all around they are told that women speak in a different voice and men have strange ways of communicating.

Are we once again to believe that anatomy is destiny? So many husbands and wives run out of patience with each other that they sometimes lose hope of ever reaching understanding. This haunting feeling of frustration is something that comes to all of us from time to time. If it helps some people to blame failures of understanding on irreconcilable gender differences, and if doing so seems to armor them against their own despair, fine. But if stereotyping serves to abstract members of the opposite sex, to turn them into categories, and to avoid genuine encounters, that is unfortunate. Exaggerating gender differences is a crutch favored by those who fail to find understanding—no, fail to *reach* understanding.

The wounded narcissism and boundless ambition of our time militate against self-sacrifice, compromise, and partnership. In hard and troubled times like ours, loyalty, tolerance, cooperation, and complementarity—the values necessary to create and sustain family harmony—are undervalued. Too often we hear what once might have been thought of as teamwork described as codependency.

We tend not to see complementarity. Instead, we see control and submission, power and weakness, villain and victim. In trying to create more flexibility for both men and women, we are in danger of forgetting that complementarity can be mutually enhancing. Self-fulfillment doesn't require constant self-assertion. The sturdy self can tolerate differences and thrive on them.

Exercises

1. Make a list of three annoying things someone in your family does on a regular basis. Next, for each one of these things, write down how you think that person would prefer to be seen. See if you can direct yourself to the person's preferred view in your next encounter. In other words, try to treat them as the people they prefer to think of themselves as.

2. Identify one boundary in your family that you don't like—for example, your wife is too involved with the children, or your husband is too distant. Remembering that boundaries are reciprocal (enmeshment in one place is related to disengagement in another), try to identify the part you play in perpetuating the boundary you don't like. Don't be in a rush to change anything; just observe.

3. Try to identify two or three triangles you participate in. If there is a triangle where you are on the uncomfortable outside, try moving not to the person you want to be closer to but to the person or activity on the other pole. For example, if you're a father who resents all the time your wife spends with the kids, try moving closer to the kids and see what happens.

4. Are you more enmeshed with or disengaged from your children? With your partner? For an experiment, try moving closer or further away and notice what signs of resistance or unbending routines block your movement.

12
. . .
From
"Do I Have *To?"*
to "That's Not Fair!"
Listening to Children and Teenagers

When new parents leave the hospital to bring home their first baby, that smiling miracle of their own creation, they wonder, *What now? How will we know what to do?* They soon find out. A baby's needs are simple, and the crying that announces them is simply overwhelming.

Once the baby is fed and changed and has had enough sleep, parents convey their responsiveness through cuddling and play. "Listening" at this age consists of reading the baby's mood—rather than imposing the parents' moods, as though the baby were an extension of themselves.

Long before a baby can talk, his parents demonstrate how well they are able to listen. Here as elsewhere, flexibility and responsiveness make for willingness to tolerate the otherness of another being. Call it sensitivity.

The Parent's Gift of Empathy

A parent's empathy—understanding what a child is feeling and showing it—builds a bridge of understanding, linking the child to someone who

252

listens and cares, thus confirming that the child's feelings are legitimate. The sharing of emotional experience is the most powerful feature of true relatedness.

How do you empathize with a child who won't stop pestering, as though he were the center of the universe and you had no concerns of your own? The solution is not to mistake sympathy for empathy. Sympathy means to feel the same as rather than to be understanding of. It's an emotion that makes people suffer *with* others, and that feeling motivates parents to talk children out of their feelings or to do *for* them rather than to empathize *with* them.

Foremost among the obstacles to listening are those that stem from our need to *do something* about what someone tells us: defend ourselves, disagree, or solve the other person's problems. Parents are prone to offer advice; it comes with the job description. But if a father's first response to his son's painful sunburn is that he should have used sunblock, the boy will feel blamed rather than commiserated with. Likewise, if a little girl complains that she doesn't have any friends and her mother tells her that if she acted friendlier, other children would be more friendly in return, the girl might conclude that even her mother doesn't like her.

Psychologists use the term *empathic immersion* to describe the intense and focused listening that therapists use to understand their patients' experience. It is an evocative metaphor, but it is of course hyperbole. Perhaps a better metaphor for empathy would be taking someone's hand.[1] Two clasped hands are still two hands—but they are also two hands touching, the warmth and pulse of one in contact with the other.

To be better listeners parents should lead less and follow more. If a child shows signs of distress, a simple statement like "You feel bad, don't you?" is more likely to make him feel understood than pressuring him to explain what he feels. If an exasperated child indicates that she wants to be alone, let her. She may need time to pull herself together. If someone is having a hard time putting something into words, it's more empathic to say "It's hard to explain, isn't it?" than to guess what the person is trying to say. A parent who finishes a child's thoughts for him is the opposite of empathic.

---

[1] I am indebted to Alfie Kohn for this metaphor. Alfie Kohn, *The Brighter Side of Human Nature: Altruism and Empathy in Everyday Life* (New York: Basic Books, 1990).

• • •

Listening well is more midwifery than dentistry.
In the presence of an empathic listener, children are able
to discover their own minds rather than having to resist
or succumb to what someone else expects them to feel.

• • •

The empathic failure that saps self-regard isn't the kind of child abuse we usually hear about; it is a silent, invidious lack of responsiveness. Empathic failure doesn't batter, bruise, or injure children; it deflates them.

Empathy is energizing. Being listened to releases us from brooding self-absorption and mobilizes us to engage the world around us. With insufficient empathy children grow up preoccupied with themselves, as though attention were a need that, unmet, keeps growing. The unlistened-to child remains locked in silent conversation within himself, too anxious and unavailable to enter the freedom of the moment.

Listening to Young Children

Being listened to creates a sense of being cared for. Not being listened to generates insecurity. In practice, not being listened to may take forms that aren't always obvious. Here are some cues that you're not listening to a young child—despite the fact that you care very much.

"Watch Out!"

Some parents who seem attentive are more concerned with the external environment than their children. They hover over their babies and make sympathetic noises, but they don't listen. They pay attention to the hard edges of a table, sharp things on the floor, cold drafts, and hot food. Because they worry a lot, they seem involved with their children. But because they're preoccupied with trying to make the world safe, they remain too anxious to share the baby's experience. These "child-centered" parents provide almost no experience of intersubjectivity. The impression of closeness they convey is an illusion. Hovered-over but not-listened-to children may become dependent, in the sense of being uneasy on their own—not because they're used to intimacy but because they suffer from a pervasive sense of aloneness, an intolerable feeling from which they use superficial relationships to distract themselves.

"Quiet Down, Go Wash Your Hands, and for Goodness' Sake, Don't Touch Yourself There!"

More common than this general lack of attunement is the selective attunement by which parents convey to their children what is shareable and what is shameful. In this way the parents' desires, fears, prohibitions, and fantasies affect the wiring of a child's self-system, leaving the child with the conviction that he is or is not a self worthy of respect.

Selective attunement determines what falls inside or outside the realm of acceptability. Is it all right to bang toys on the floor, to get dirty, to touch yourself? It includes preferences for people: is it all right to get mad at Grandma or sometimes to prefer to play with her rather than with Mommy? And it includes the extent to which internal states—joy, sadness, delight—can be experienced with another person. Is the child whose parents try to jolly him out of it when he's frightened likely to come to them with his fears when he's older?

It's the breadth of attunement—from generous to cramped—that determines whether children feel okay about themselves and whether they have a broad or narrow range of experience.

Suppose a toddler listening to *Peter and the Wolf* is happy and excited. He's moved by the music and wonders if his mother feels it too. He looks up, and she smiles back at him; her eyes are bright and she's nodding. *Yes, she feels it too!* With this attunement, the child knows that he is feeling something that can be shared—rather than something that should be stifled. His feeling is validated; and since the feeling is part of him, he too is validated.

"Don't Brag. It's Not Nice."

In addition to the lessons parents teach deliberately, they shape their children's experience with negative affective responses. When a child proudly shows off to a parent who responds with disgust or disinterest, it's a slap in the face of the child's healthy narcissism. This is shame.

What children show off for their parents' approval isn't simply what they can do; it's also their fantasies of who they wish they were and what they dream of doing. They're not little and weak—oh no, they're big and strong! If parents squelch that wonderful wish to make an impression, the child may decide that he's unworthy or that he has to achieve really big things for anybody to notice.

Before you let negative reactions slip out, think about why you're tempted to be so critical or disapproving. Is it really a prohibition your child needs, or are you more concerned about what other people might think? Sometimes, in an attempt to instill social graces too early, we crush a child's self-esteem. *Listen* to what your child is saying. The little girl who shouts, "I can jump higher than Robbie!" isn't putting down her friend; she's seeking your approval. Why not give it to her?

Are your admonitions based on trying to force a child to live up to your own expectations? A little girl runs to her mother and says, "Mommy, Mommy, guess what! I got an A in spelling!" "That's nice, dear," the mother responds, sounding pleased, but not very. The daughter tries again. "There's *twenty-nine* kids, and I got the second highest score." "That's good, honey." The conversation continues for another couple of minutes, with the little girl, proud and excited, trying to drive up her mother's enthusiasm, and the mother pleased that her daughter did well but not wanting her to get hooked on achievement (like her father). When the little girl persists, the mother finally says, "Don't brag. It isn't nice."

One minute the little girl is throbbing with excitement. Getting an A was wonderful. She rushed home to tell her mother to complete her experience. You could say she met with misunderstanding, but it was worse. Because a child seeking appreciation is reaching out, exposed, a failed response is an emotional head-on collision.

Empathic failure can come out sounding mean: "Don't be such a baby!" "Stop showing off!" But even a simple lack of enthusiasm can hurt a child who's eager for attention. When our children make the mistake of daring not to be invented by us, when they reveal, perversely, minds and wills of their own, we are put to the test.

"Why Must You Argue with Everything I Say!"

Few things are more exasperating to parents than constant arguing. "Do I have to?" "It's not fair!" "I don't want to!" and, of course, "Why? Why? Why?" Who wants to listen to that all day?

The best way to defuse arguments is to separate the *expressive* function of communication from the *instrumental*. Let children complain. Show your understanding by listening. It shouldn't be too hard to listen if you have the final say. Unfortunately, the usual formula—"I understand, but … "—doesn't work very well. It isn't paraphrasing what children say or telling them that you understand that makes them feel taken seriously; it's letting them express themselves. It's listening.

Responsive listening works by drawing children out, encouraging them to talk about what they want, and, if feasible, postponing any decision until later. The more children are encouraged to express themselves, and the more this part of the dialogue is separated from laying down the law, the more children are likely to accept what they're told to do.

What's the Best Way to Disarm Children's Resistance to Doing What They're Told?

The answer is, you don't disarm a child's resistance—you accept it as a perfectly legitimate expression of the child's feelings.

Children deserve to have their feelings taken seriously. What they don't need are elaborate explanations. The well-meaning attempt to explain to a four-year-old *why* she has to go to bed is misguided. Explaining such decisions implies that they have to be justified—and are therefore open to debate. It's different with teenagers. Explaining the rules to teenagers shows respect for their maturing status. Younger children don't need to know why their parents have rules; they need to know that their parents are in charge.

Whining[2]

When little children don't get what they want, they whine. They beg and they plead, and they keep at it until they get their way or drive their parents up the wall.

---

[2]Much of the material in this section is taken from my book *Stop Arguing with Your Kids* (New York: Guilford Press, 2004).

• • •

**Everyone knows that giving in to whining doesn't work.
And they're wrong.**

• • •

Giving in to whining works very well, actually. Giving in stops the fussing (and reinforces the child for doing so). What's more, the parent is reinforced for giving in—by the child's quieting down. Psychologists call this *negative reinforcement*. Positive reinforcement increases behavior by rewarding it. Giving a pigeon a pellet for pressing a bar and giving a whining child a cookie are both examples of positive reinforcement. Negative reinforcement works by removing an unpleasant stimulus. A pigeon's pressing a bar to turn off a blast of air and a parent's giving in to a whining child to make him quiet down are both examples of negative reinforcement.

Child psychologists recommend that parents refuse to be manipulated by whining. The most effective strategy is to ignore it. No response, no reinforcement. If whining occurs in public, don't scold or argue. Just remove the child from the scene. The lesson is, whining leads to exclusion.

If whining occurs at home, parents are advised to pay no attention. They should just go about their business without lecturing or fussing. Lecturing and fussing constitute the other half of an argument. Ignoring a whining child means not only not debating with the child but also not sighing or giving angry looks. These nonverbal signals are also responses, and they prolong whining every bit as much as scolding.

If you want to eliminate whining, ignoring it is good advice. The best way to diminish any form of behavior is not to respond to it. But do you really just want to eliminate your child's whining?

Whining becomes manipulative, but it doesn't start out that way. It starts as an expression of the child's feelings. By using responsive listening you can tune in to a whining child's feelings and shift the interaction from a struggle to a conversation.

• • •

**Whining is a request for attention. If you stop and focus
on the child—"What are you trying to say, honey?"—
the whining will usually stop.**

• • •

Alice was trying to talk with her mother about finding a nursing home for her father. Four-year-old Amy kept interrupting—perhaps she sensed her mother's anxiety—and Alice told her to go and play. The interruptions continued until, finally losing her temper, Alice spanked Amy and sent her to bed.

Alternatively: Alice was trying to talk with her mother about finding a nursing home for her father. Four-year-old Amy kept interrupting—perhaps she sensed her mother's anxiety—and Alice told her to go and play. When that didn't work, Alice bent down and picked Amy up and said, "What's the matter honey?"

"How come I never get to talk to Grandma?" Amy asked.

"I know, honey, you want to visit with Grandma." Then she took Amy by the hand and walked with her over to her toys and said, "In ten minutes, you can take Grandma outside and show her your swing set."

Children don't whine just to be annoying. They have legitimate concerns. They whine because they're unable to express themselves in a more mature way. They're frustrated. They're tired. They're young. The parent who responds punitively—"Stop that noise!"—is inadvertently supplying the other half of the argument. The parent who ignores a whining child conveys—"I won't listen to you when you're upset." Or, worse, "I won't listen to you until you get *really* upset."

Tantrums

Whining escalates to tantrums when children give up asking for what they want and give in to frustration. Now, instead of pleading their case, children start kicking and screaming.

The child who throws a tantrum may be trying to get his way, but he's become too upset to put his feelings into words. In responding to a child in the throes of a tantrum, the principles of responsive listening still apply, but you must take into account the child's loss of control. First and foremost, don't respond to a child's tantrum with an argument. Don't repeat what made the child upset in the first place—"I said no, and I meant it!"— and never tell a child who's having a tantrum to calm down.

• • •

**Telling a child who's upset to calm down implies
that she has no right to her feelings.**

• • •

When dealing with a child who's having a tantrum, remember that an argument is a tug of war:

"Yes, you will!"

"No, I won't!"

Avoid escalating the argument by continuing to verbally oppose the child—"I don't care what you do; I'm not going to change my mind!"—and don't tell the child to control himself. Instead, begin by trying to acknowledge what the child is feeling. Since he's probably too upset to put his feelings into words, help him.

"Wow, you're really mad, aren't you?"

Notice that putting this statement in the form of a question invites the child to agree. This may not be a good idea. Inviting someone to agree leaves open the possibility of arguing. A better alternative is to reflect what the child seems to be feeling without asking him to agree.

"Wow, you're really mad!"

What I'm suggesting here may seem like an exception to the rule of helping people to elaborate their feelings with a question. How does saying "Wow, you're really mad!" qualify as responsive listening?

The essence of responsive listening is *permission giving*. The idea is to give children permission to feel what they feel and to express those feelings to someone who cares. The reason for not asking children in the throes of a tantrum questions about their feelings is that they're too overwrought to explain. Here a reflection of feelings lets the child know that you understand—and gives him permission to elaborate or disagree if he wishes.

Most accurate reflections of feeling are punctuated with an exclamation point. Try saying out loud, "Wow, you're really mad." Then say the same thing with an exclamation point. See the difference? Oops, I mean: What a difference!

Reflecting a tantruming child's feelings won't magically make him calm down. What it will do is let him know that you understand what he's feeling and, more important, it will avoid the tug of war of trying to argue with a child who's out of control.

Speaking Up for Themselves

From five to twelve, children spend a lot of time learning the rules. They learn to conform to the expectations of teachers and principals and lunch room ladies and bus drivers and soccer coaches and Scout leaders and Sunday school teachers—and, of course, their parents. Parents of school-age children have to make sure their kids get ready for school in the morning, do their homework at night, put away their clothes, do their chores, turn off the computer, don't kill their brothers and sisters, brush their teeth, and get ready for bed on time. Arguments become the rule.

Some adults respond to children's challenging the rules as though it were an attack on themselves. Authoritarian parents and teachers expect to be obeyed without question. Arguments are an affront to their authority. A child who argues for more flexibility may have no intention of challenging anyone's authority. He or she is just wants more freedom. But if adults insist that respecting their authority means obeying without question, then children are forced to disrespect them in order to challenge the rules. Thus, whether children's speaking up for themselves is seen as a legitimate form of self-expression or an attack depends on how adults interpret it.

Standing up for what you want isn't the same as being disrespectful. If parents and teachers respect children's rights to argue, the children will respect their right to decide. But children whose feelings aren't accepted as legitimate will turn from arguing their points to challenging your right to control them. Show respect for children by listening to what they have to say, even when it's inconvenient.

In studying the families of five- to twelve-year-old children, researchers found that encouraging give-and-take was associated with skill in communication, while parents with an authoritarian style ("Because I said so!") who discouraged responses from their children produced higher levels of verbal aggressiveness.[3] The take-home lesson is that listening is a two-way street.

● ● ●

The single most important thing you can do to develop a cooperative relationship is to listen to what your child has to say. Once children have had a chance to say what's on their minds—and have their feelings acknowledged— they become more receptive to what you have to say.

● ● ●

If a child doesn't do what he or she agreed to, don't nag; find out why.

"I notice that you didn't show me your homework like you said you would."

"I forgot."

"Maybe there's a reason you forgot. Is it that you hate doing homework, or do you not like having to show it to me?"

Sustaining Empathy as Children Grow

Thinking about sad-faced children, it's hard not to be touched. You want to put your arms around those kids and love them. You know how they feel. But here's where it's possible to get confused. Empathy is generous, and so it's easy to slide into thinking of it as just another way of saying loving kindness. Empathy is loving, but it doesn't mean being affectionate or supportive or helpful or a lot of other nice things. Some parents are loving, but the love they express is so suffocating that it smothers their children's initiative and is anything but empathic.

● ● ●

It's easier to listen to children's wants when parents are firm with their wills.

● ● ●

---

[3]Cherie L. Bayer and Donald J. Cegala, "Trait Verbal Aggressiveness and Argumentativeness: Relations with Parenting Style," *Western Journal of Communication*, 1992, 56, 301–310.

Parents who allow the boundary between generations to erode become not grownups-in-charge but peers and playmates, without the authority to enforce boundaries or the credibility to comfort and protect. "No" is less palatable than "yes," and so it's often served with a lot of verbal sauce, the way some people try to get kids to eat vegetables by smothering them in butter and salt (the vegetables). These parents won't magically take charge if someone teaches them to use gold stars and time-out chairs. Setting limits and enforcing rules—beginning when children are small—follows naturally from maintaining a clear boundary between the generations. It also permits and facilitates empathy.

When children are little, the greatest impediment to empathy is a parent's not being in charge. When children get a little older, the hardest part of empathy is letting them be themselves. Most parents can empathize with children when they're little. They're comfortable with closeness. But sustaining empathy means allowing children to differentiate, to have their own wishes, their own interests, their own feelings. Children aren't merely cute or headstrong; they're people, and they yearn, like you and me, to be taken seriously.

Perhaps the most important shift a parent can make is to move from wanting their children to be successful to being pleased with them, right now, loving them, enjoying them, and accepting that they are who they are. They are separate from us; they are themselves. Parents can begin to really hear their children only when they set aside thinking of them as unfinished products, clay for the parents to mold. None of this is meant to say that we shouldn't limit our children's behavior—for our own convenience as well as for their own good. But once we accept that they are who they are, for better or worse, we can worry less about them, relax our attempts to control and reform and manipulate and improve them, and concentrate on listening to them.

Listening to Teenagers

One reason parenting remains an amateur sport is that as soon as you get the hang of it, the children get a little older and throw you a whole new set of curves. Wise parents learn to shift their style of parenting to accommodate to their children's development.

Marlene could hardly believe that her little boy was fifteen. It didn't seem that long ago that Dylan had followed her around the house wanting to do everything with her. Now he was a gangly adolescent who wanted nothing to do with her. Almost overnight, it seemed, her little boy had shot up, sprouted hair on his face, and developed an attitude.

Dylan still occasionally tolerated his mother's company, but even then he could be hard to talk to. One minute they'd be chatting amiably, and the next thing you knew Dylan would lapse into gloomy silence.

Dylan didn't argue with his parents openly, the way many teenagers did, but he was getting harder to talk to. Half the time all he seemed to do was grunt.

Adolescence is a famously difficult time for the family. Most teenagers go through a period of rebelliousness, defining themselves as independent through opposition to their parents. Some fight openly with their parents; others, like Dylan, go underground.

If we look at the family as a system in transformation, we can see teenagers in the vanguard for change. In pushing for autonomy they want to loosen the ties that hold them back and redefine their relationship with their parents. Conflict is inevitable because, while parents want to slow the transition ("I'm still your father"), teenagers want to speed it up ("Don't you trust me?").

Early signs of defiance begin at age twelve or thirteen. Preadolescents begin to argue about everything—baggy pants, short skirts, tattoos, eating habits, chores, messy rooms, homework, cell phones, computer time, television, R-rated movies, parties. It's tempting to say that the outcome of these struggles depends on the quality of communication between parents and children. And while to a certain extent that's true, the underlying issue is attitudinal.

The problem isn't just curfews or clothes; the real problem is that teenagers are challenging the rules that govern family relationships. They no longer want to be treated like children. They want to be treated like people.

As parents, we tend to see things through the prism of our own experience. We weren't as advantaged as today's teens. We didn't have cell phones or computers. Our parents didn't spend the kind of money on us that we spend on our kids. Today's teenagers have it easy. All they have to do is stand by while their bodies, raging with hormones, shoot up, change shape, and sprout hair in the most unlikely places. Well, not exactly stand by—just finish high school, figure out what they want to do with the rest of their lives, get good grades, do volunteer work, fall in love and have their hearts broken, make friends, lose friends, and transform themselves from the children they were to the adults they want to be. How hard can that be?

Adolescence is almost inevitably a difficult passage for the whole family, but it needn't be as antagonistic as we've come to expect. It can be an enjoyable, even exciting, time for everyone in the family. Teenagers bring new styles, new attitudes, and new information into the family. They keep their parents up to date and on their toes. Although some parents get defensive and resist their children's changing status, others welcome the breath of fresh ideas.

Holding On and Letting Go

Parents can err in either of two directions: by letting their children go too early and too easily, thus depriving them of support and guidance; or by holding on too tight, too long, and thus becoming a force against which to rebel. Flexible boundaries give teenagers room to explore but keep lines of communication open. What's the secret of finding the right balance? Listening works wonders.

But it's not just listening as a passive taking in. It's making an active effort to tune in and hear what your teenager is saying. It's connecting.

"My Kids Never Talk to Me Anymore."

"How was school today?"

"Fine."

"What are you doing?"

"Nothing."

One of the hardest things about being a parent of teenagers is that they start to shut you out. Beginning at about age eleven some kids begin to slip away from their parents, retreating more and more into their own worlds. By fourteen most teenagers are a mystery to their parents.

Teenagers don't talk to their parents because they don't expect to get listened to. Would you open up to someone if you anticipated criticism, interrogation, and advice giving?

Don't Pry

The quickest way to get shut out is to ask prying questions. Spend time with your kids, but be patient; wait for the oyster to open.

Adolescence is a time of exquisite sensitivity to criticism because it's not just an emerging self but a changing self that is vulnerable to acceptance or rejection. Exposed and trapped in their own bodies, preoccupied and troubled about sex, popularity, achievement, success, self-indulgence, and self-denial, teenagers are on display all day at school and they feel under terrific scrutiny. No wonder they're sensitive to what their parents say.

• • •

Whether or not children open up to their parents depends on the reception they expect.

• • •

Teenagers won't open up to their parents if they expect their feelings to be disavowed.

"It can't be that bad."

"You're making too much out of it."

"Nobody is that mean."

"You must have done something to make him respond that way."

It isn't just words that convey this lack of acceptance; it can be changing the subject, rolling your eyes, or ignoring your teenager's feelings altogether.

What do teenagers do when they stay out late? Most parents would love to know. But when they ask too many questions, they get few answers, because kids don't like to be cross-examined.

"What did you do?"

"Who was there?"

"Why did you do that?"

"What were you doing there in the first place?"

These same parents may complain that their teenagers don't share with them what's going on with their friends or at school.

"Did you have fun today?"

"Why do you stay in your room?"

"Why aren't you going to the dance?"

"Do any of your friends take drugs?"

"What's wrong with asking questions?" you ask. Nothing. It's not so much the questions that turn teenagers off; it's that parents ask their children to reveal their feelings but don't reveal any of their own. This feels like an interrogation, rather than a mutual exchange.

What Happens When Your Kids Talk to You?

Did that question make you think about what your kids do in conversation with you? How about what you do?

Do you give them your full attention? Do you turn off the TV or computer? Do you put down the paper? Do you make eye contact?

If you give your children half of your attention, what are you telling them they're worth to you?

Oh, you do give your kids your full attention? In fact, you're dying to get them to talk to you? But do you approach them with an open, receptive attitude? Are you prepared to hear what's on their minds, or do you pressure them to talk about what's on your mind?

Another form of teenage withholding is "silent arguing."

Todd walked into the living room where his son Daniel was sprawled on the couch watching TV. "Danny," he said, "tomorrow is garbage day. Will you please take out the garbage before you go to bed?"

"Uh-huh," Daniel replied.

The following evening when Todd came home from work, he was annoyed to see the garbage bag still sitting in the kitchen where he'd left it the night before. He was annoyed, not only because the garbage hadn't been taken out, but also because Daniel had broken yet another agreement with him.

As should be obvious, Todd didn't really have an agreement with his son. He asked Daniel to do something while he was watching TV, and Daniel mumbled whatever it would take to get his father to leave him alone. Daniel probably didn't intend *not* to take out the garbage, but he never really made a conscious commitment to do so.

Although some teenagers don't argue openly with their parents, they don't exactly do what they're asked, either. They agree only to avoid being hassled. Their "okay" doesn't mean "Okay, I'll do it" as much as "Okay, I hear you, now leave me alone."

Silent Arguing

You can recognize silent arguing in a pattern of a teenager's not doing what you expect of him or her and with a general avoidance of discussion. When confronted, the silent arguer will say "I forgot" or "Okay, I'll do it later."

When someone repeatedly fails to do what you expect, it's a safe bet that he or she doesn't want to. That much may be obvious. But what may be less obvious is that silent arguers often "forget" because they don't think something really needs to be done or they don't think it's fair that they have to be the one to do it. One way to find out is to ask.

● ● ●

The reason for silent arguing is not believing that the other person is open to your point of view.

● ● ●

"It seems like I always have to remind you to cut the grass. Do you resent having to do it?"

"Do you think it isn't fair that I want you to make your bed in the morning?"

"I'm guessing there's a good reason you never seem to get around to doing your homework. Believe it or not, I'm really interested in how you feel about it."

In business dealings, responsive listening is a powerful tool for overcoming resistance. If you want to convince somebody of something, the best strategy is first to get him to express all the reasons he's reluctant to. Once you've heard his reservations, they no longer operate as an unspoken barrier to hearing your ideas.

You can use the same strategy to help overcome resistance from your kids. But do you really want to deal with your children as though strategizing to outwit an adversary? Or do you genuinely want to hear what your kids think? And are you willing to take their ideas about what's fair into account?

In studying what adolescent girls value most in their relationships with their mothers, researchers found that daughters appreciate their mothers listening to their ideas, mothers sharing their own feelings, and relationships changing as a result of give and take. Daughters were much more willing to listen to their mothers' suggestions after having had a chance to express their own opinions.[4]

While some teenagers describe their parents as bossy, they also describe themselves as stubborn: "We don't like to admit that the other is right. I go, She might be right and I may believe what she is saying, but I won't say it."[5]

It is this readiness to resist control that responsive listening is designed to overcome. Teenagers are more likely to cooperate with agreements that they've had a hand in negotiating. But if parents aren't really willing to

---

[4]Carol Gilligan, Nona Lyons, and Trudy Hanmer, eds., *Making Connections: The Relational Worlds of Adolescent Girls at Emma Willard School* (Cambridge, MA: Harvard University Press, 1990).

[5]Gilligan, Lyons, and Hanmer, p. 265.

compromise, teenagers soon see "negotiations" for what they are: a sham, just another parents' trick for imposing their will.

> "You can't go ice skating on Sunday if you haven't finished your homework for Monday."

> This isn't a contract. There was no negotiation.

> "If you want to go ice skating, what do you propose doing about your homework?"

> "I'll do it after I come home."

> "By the time you get home from the skating rink, it'll be time for supper."

> "Okay. How about if I finish all my homework before we go skating. Then can I go?"

> "Sure, that's fine."

Why go to all the trouble to come up with such an obvious solution? Because the child came up with it. If the parent had imposed it, the teenager would feel resentful and be less motivated to live up to it.

When discussions turn into quarrels, the parent who uses responsive listening is way ahead of the game. But knowing when to switch from negotiating to just listening—and remaining cool enough to do so—can be extremely difficult. A better strategy is to be proactive instead of reactive. Instead of waiting for disagreements to crop up, parents can circumvent a lot of arguments by initiating discussions about family rules before they become problems.

Set aside time to be with your children and encourage them to bring up requests and complaints. This kind of initiation produces a whole different atmosphere.

Avoiding Battles for Control

It's often said that today's children don't respect authority. They argue with their parents and speak rudely to their teachers. Who teaches children to argue? Adults who get into needless battles for control.

"I'm Not a Morning Person."

1. *Dog whistle*: a high-pitched instrument that human beings can't hear.

2. *Alarm clock*: a medium-pitched instrument that teenagers can't hear.

3. *Parents*: see definition #2.

"You're Right."

Most people understand that adolescent rebellion is normal, but as adults we tend to interpret children's experience primarily in relation to ourselves. Parents who think of their teenagers as "defiant" confuse autonomous strivings with stubbornness. Most teenagers are strong-willed, not oppositional. They struggle not to defy their parents but to gain respect and freedom. How far they carry that struggle, how extreme their behavior, is determined largely by how tenaciously parents resist recognizing their voice in an effort to retain control.

Too many parents are afraid to say "You're right." They're afraid that letting their children be right makes them wrong and afraid that letting the children win means that the parents will lose. In fact, the opposite is true.

A girl who can't win control of how to dress for school may seek to express herself by putting on dramatic makeup after she leaves the house. If she can't win that battle, she may escalate the conflict further, deliberately coming home late or getting into shouting matches with her mother. Or she may defy her parents by smoking cigarettes or shoplifting or experimenting with drugs. Reckless experiments, chancy relationships—all for the honor of proving she has some say in her life. Wouldn't it be easier to give it to her?

• • •

What makes responsive listening with teenagers hard is that they are no longer grateful just to have their feelings acknowledged. Now they expect their opinions to be considered.

• • •

A frequent complaint of teenagers is that their parents don't listen to them. Teenagers are exquisitely sensitive to disrespect; they want to be treated like people with a right to their opinions. Often without realizing, parents provoke adolescents by talking to them from the same one-up position they used when the children were small. The "rude" response is a protest against what feels like a put-down. Parents can avoid escalating arguments into power struggles by tolerating their children's right to say whatever they think, even if it means using language parents don't like.

Don't Take the Bait

How do you avoid being provoked by a teenager's cracks? The same way a fish avoids getting hooked. By not rising to the bait.

Not rising to the bait is, of course, easier said than done when you're dealing with virtuosos of the put-down. It's a skill teenagers develop sparring with their friends, where they learn to protect themselves by cutting other people down to size. But when teenagers use mockery with their parents, they don't always say what they mean.

What They Say	Translation
"Whatever—."	"That's stupid and I wish you'd drop it."
"Chill out."	"Don't get so upset; you're acting like a fool."
"Okay, Mom."	Politer version of "whatever," meaning, basically, "Leave me alone."
"Yeah, sure, Dad."	"That's ridiculous, and you're an idiot."
Sarcastic look	"You are beneath contempt. But I don't dare tell you what I think."

It's hard to defend yourself against these zingers because they rarely cross the double line. Why don't teenagers say what they mean? Because they're afraid of how their parents will respond.

What do you do when your teenager gets snotty with you? You can counterattack, you can walk away, or you can talk about it.[6] The most direct thing you say when somebody hurts you is "That hurts." But remem-

---

[6] I favor strategy number two. When somebody hurts my feelings, I walk away. I get very quiet, and I stay that way for two or three days. This strategy, technically known as pouting, must be a good one because I learned it back in the good old days, when I was about four.

ber, you're the parent. You can do more than avoid fighting back. You can use responsive listening to find out what's behind your teenager's sarcastic comments.

"Do you feel I've been unfair?"

"What do I do that makes you feel like treating me like that?"

You'll have to convince your child that you're really willing to hear the answer to such questions. Parents who are willing to listen to their children even when it's hard are better able to handle the inevitable battles with their teenagers.

Recognizing Their Need to Break Away

A major reason for lack of communication between teenagers and parents is the parents' failure to accept the inevitable: if children are to grow up, they must break away from the older generation. It's a teenager's job to criticize his parents. The same children who once looked up to Mommy and Daddy as giants who can do no wrong now look down on them as old fogies who can do nothing right. This disdainful attitude is a natural stage in the evolution of the family and the development of the self. It's a necessary part of becoming your own person.

It may not be pleasant to hear teenagers criticizing everything and everybody, but it's part of the process of building self-esteem. Parents who criticize their children for being critical are fighting fire with gasoline.

The more inflexible parents are, the more defiant teenagers will be. Too many put-downs wear away at children's self-esteem and prompt them to reject their parents. Some people are so ashamed of their parents that they spend their whole lives trying not to be like them. They're so busy *not being* their parents that there's no room left for them to be themselves.

In the process of looking for new models of how to be, teenagers often glom onto someone outside the family—it can be almost anyone, just as long as he or she is different, and perhaps more willing than the parents to take the child seriously. When this happens, their ability to hear their parents is compromised, though they may have a fairness channel that remains open. If a parent can listen calmly and demonstrate openness to what a teenager is trying to say, but the child doesn't reciprocate, the parent can say, "You're not being fair to me." The child may then listen. Teenagers respect fairness, especially if it is reciprocal.

Breaking Out of Mutual Antagonism

One reason parents and teenagers have trouble getting through to each other is that each side hears the other only as objects in relation to themselves. When teenagers, who want respect and freedom, come to expect only criticism and control, they shut their ears to what their parents are trying to say and respond reflexively with either resistance or passive compliance. It's not just the interactions between parents and children that result in conflict; it's the way they interpret those interactions.

> "I'm sorry I yelled at her, but she has absolutely no respect for anything I say."

> "Okay, I lied. But my parents never let me do anything."

When parents come to think of their teenagers as "defiant," they develop tunnel vision, which leads them to notice and remember only those events that fit the Defiant Teenager story line. Thus, a father who comes to see his son as "selfish" and "irresponsible" will remember the times his son didn't do his chores or was caught drinking beer and tend to forget the times when his son volunteered to mow the lawn or helped cook supper. Each of the son's transgressions confirms the father's story line that his son doesn't really live up to his responsibilities. The son, in turn, may be acutely aware of the times his father refuses to give him a ride to the mall or let him go to a party with his friends. Thus, he gradually develops a narrative around never being able to satisfy his father, which makes him give up caring what his father thinks. Both father and son remain stuck in a cycle, not simply of control and defiance but, more specifically, of noticing only incidents of control or defiance.

Such closed and rigid narratives make parents and teenagers reactive to each other and quick to argue.

Marcia's fifteen-year-old son Jonathan wanted to spend the night at the home of a friend whom the parents haven't met.

"I don't want you sleeping over at someone's house that we don't know. You should know better than to ask." Marcia defended her decision with indignation, as though her son's request was another example of his selfish disregard for any reasonable set of expectations.

Jonathan's face reddened. He'd been ready for a fight, and sure enough, here it was. "Why not!" he demanded. "I'll bring him over here after school, so that you can meet him if that's so important to you." It didn't matter what Marcia said in response. Whatever reasons his mother gave, Jonathan was prepared to shoot down.

Marcia, who didn't really have any reasons and was now too mad at this latest incident of her son's "rudeness," could only sputter, "Because I don't want you to, that's why."

"Mom! What the hell—you're so unreasonable!"

"Leave me alone. I'm tired," Marcia said, her cheeks blotched with color. "Because I don't want you springing things on me at the last minute. That's all."

"Why can't I see my friends!" Jonathan moaned. "I don't want to be here!"

Notice how this argument is driven by "totalizing views"—mother and son reducing each other to one set of frustrating responses. Jonathan wasn't mad just because his mother wouldn't let him sleep over at his friend's house. He was mad because his mother *Never Lets Him Do Anything*. His mother is *Totally Unfair*. Aren't all parents?

Likewise, Marcia wasn't upset just because Jonathan wanted to sleep over at his friend's house. She was angry because her son is *Rude*. He's *Selfish*, *Demanding*, *Disrespectful*. Aren't all teenagers?

Parents reduce their children to stereotypes when they focus only on the things that disappoint them. The child who doesn't do what you want is, by definition, stubborn, right? Parents who see their teenagers as "stubborn" and "irresponsible," as though that were the sum total of their being, are likely to be seen in turn as "unfair" and "demanding." When this happens, both sides collect grievances, saving them up like coupons. For what?

Is the common parental view of teenagers as "lazy" a complete distortion? No, a lot of teenagers are lazy around the house. That's because home is the natural arena for expressing the dependent, childish part of themselves. The teenager's more independent and considerate side is usually on view only away from home, often unseen by his parents.

What's the Matter with That Kid?

When teenagers seem to be acting unreasonably, it may help to consider what view of their parents would make those actions seem reasonable.

Find a time when you're both relaxed and ask the teenager, "Do you see me as ... ?" If the teenager is brave enough to give you an honest answer, try saying: "I'm sorry. Maybe I need to work on that."

We've seen how adolescent rebelliousness is related to parental control and how control-and-rebel cycles are driven by the tendency of both generations to view each other in oppositional stereotypes. Thus, we've gone from blaming conflicts with teenagers on their rebelliousness to seeing these struggles as part of an interpersonal pattern, first in behavioral terms and then, adding a cognitive dimension, by recognizing that people's actions are based on their perceptions.

"Dad, please, can't I borrow the car? I promise to be home by 10:30."

His father was just about to say no when he paused for a moment, remembering what it was like to be a teenage boy needing a car on a Saturday night. And, with a greater empathic grasp of what it was like to be a teenage boy, he cried out, "Oh, my God!" and handcuffed his son to the bedpost.

Breaking out of the fixed narratives that fuel antagonism is difficult but not impossible. The way to break the grip of totalizing views is to ask yourself how does the other person prefer to think of himself or herself? How does he or she prefer to be seen? Once you start thinking this way, you begin to see other people's actions in a more reasonable light.

A Certain Amount of Control

You don't eliminate conflicts with adolescents just by listening to their point of view. You only win by being willing to lose a little. Or to put it another way, only by giving up on the idea of complete control can parents retain a certain amount of control over their teenagers. And, with teenagers, *a certain amount of control* is all you can hope for.

Those things that parents absolutely don't want their kids doing—smoking, drinking, having sex, cutting school, hanging around with bad company—most teenagers are going to experiment with no matter what their parents say. Actually, it's a little more complicated than that.

The adolescent's parents are already a part of him or her, in the form of a developing conscience. It is this inner voice that now begins to exert the most powerful influence on an adolescent's decisions—but not if parents are controlling or punitive. Teenagers think about what's right or wrong only when they don't have somebody standing over them telling them what to do.

Striking a Balance Between Autonomy and Connection

For all their opposition to their parents and breathless enthusiasm for the adventures of adulthood, teenagers still need their families.

Adolescents need their parents to listen to their troubles, their hopes and ambitions, even some of their far-fetched plans. The more tolerant parents are, the more they remain open to hearing their children, the more possible it is to preserve connection.

"I'm thinking about not going to college."

(After counting to ten, in Roman numerals) "That's interesting. What are you thinking about doing?"

In realizing that they can disagree and argue with their parents, adolescents come to differentiate between conventional views of family life—as nonconflicted—and a more realistic view, namely, that conflict and confrontation, and working through differences, are part of a healthy relationship.

Teenage boys still expect to be supported and understood by their parents, but perhaps more than anything else they want the freedom to be independent. Teenage girls, on the other hand, often have more complex and ambivalent relationships, especially with their mothers. As a member of Carol Gilligan's study of the relational world of adolescent girls,

Sharon Rich found that mothers' dependence on their daughters troubles the daughters and makes it harder for mothers to accept daughters' independence. Daughters want mothers to be there for them, but also to trust them, accept their independence, and honor their choices. Over and over, girls reported being unhappy with mothers they described as poor listeners.

"These girls depict themselves as receiving two messages when they feel their mothers are not listening: Their mothers do not care and are not 'there' for them; and their own opinions are not important."

As one girl in the study reflected: "I sort of feel that I don't want her to know too much about me. I mean not that I'm trying to keep everything a secret, but just that I want to be more myself and less her trying to mold me. And so there are lots of things I don't tell her because I just know what she would say ... and I don't feel like hearing it."[7]

Adolescents who don't feel listened to flare up in angry resentment, and later retreat into silence and secrecy as the best way they know to protect their vulnerable, distinct voices and themselves. In attempting to protect themselves from feeling "terrible," teenagers may cut off the primary means for improving the relationship: communication.

Unheard adolescents who flee their families are seldom really free. Protective distance affords them the illusion of being grown up, but it's only an illusion.

*   *   *

Most families have problems not because there's something wrong with them but because they've gotten stuck. Families resist change even more than individuals because the structure that holds them together is supported by the actions of every single family member. That's why systems are stubborn. What we mustn't forget, though, is that even though families act like systems, it's still individual persons who do the acting—and they, as you may have noticed, can sometimes be pretty courageous.

---

[7]Sharon Rich, "Daughters' Views of Their Relationships with Their Mothers," in Carol Gilligan, Nona Lyons, and Trudy Hanmer, eds., *Making Connections: The Relational World of Adolescent Girls at Emma Willard School* (Cambridge, MA: Harvard University Press, 1990), p. 268.

Exercises

1. Get a notebook and for one week write down every time you make a critical comment to your child. That's all. Just notice. If you have more than one child, keep a separate tally for each. Make sure you count comments that start out positive but end up negative. "I appreciate your doing the dishes, but I wish you'd remember to rinse off the soap next time."

   Notice what effect changing from positive to negative comments has on the communication between you and your child. Does he or she talk to you more when you make positive comments? Listen to you more?

2. Pick out one thing that your child fails to do consistently despite frequent reminders. Find a time when you're both relaxed to talk with the child and say that you bet he or she has a good reason for not doing that something—maybe the child doesn't think it's fair for him or her to have to—and that you'd like to hear how the child feels about it. If you're lucky enough to have your child open up, just listen. Don't end the conversation by laying down the law.

3. What were the two worst things that happened to you when you were a teenager? Did you tell your parents? Why did you or didn't you tell them? What were the consequences?

4. Think of a conflict a parent might have with a teenager. Write down something a parent might say that fits into each of the following categories:

Criticism	Accusing
Lecturing	Orders
Threats	Lecturing
Comparisons	Moralizing
Name-calling	Sarcasm
Shaming	Prophecies of doom
Blaming	Martyrdom

5. For a few days, keep track of your interactions with your children. Estimate the percentage of time you spend listening versus the percentage of time you spend talking.

   If your kids don't seem to want to talk with you, it's all their fault. See? You're off the hook.

13

...

"I Knew You'd Understand"

Being Able to Hear Friends and Colleagues

Friends make the best listeners. They may not love us quite as much as our families do, but then they don't need quite as much from us either, and that frees them to listen better. No matter how close we are to our friends, we retain a certain independence, which enables us to listen without needing to control them or protect ourselves.

Why Friends Make the Best Listeners

Sandy had just come from a workshop on counseling high school students when she met her friend Roberta for lunch. If she didn't trust Roberta's support so completely, Sandy might have hesitated to tell her that she was thinking about doing something that would mean an end to their lunches. The two of them had been teaching French at the same school for nine years, and now Sandy had decided to go back and get a master's in guidance counseling. It was a big decision, scary and exciting, and she needed someone to talk it over with.

Roberta was taken aback by Sandy's plan. Giving up tenure and going back to school seemed risky. How did Sandy know she would like counseling? Wasn't she taking a big chance? Besides, Roberta couldn't imagine getting along at work without her friend. Sandy was the only sane person in the place. It would be awful if she left. But Roberta didn't say any of this. No matter how much she questioned Sandy's plan, it was her decision, and Roberta could see how excited she was by this new dream of hers. So she just listened.

It took Sandy two more days to get up the nerve to mention going back to school to her husband. "I can't believe you'd even think of such a thing!" Gordon said. "Are you crazy? You've got a perfectly good job. How are we going to pay for you to go to school?" Sandy started to protest, but she was too hurt to bother, and they finished supper in silence.

Roberta's ability to listen to Sandy was the mirror opposite of her husband's inability. Roberta could listen because she wasn't threatened—or at least not *as* threatened.

Clearly Gordon had a stake in whether or not Sandy went back to school. He had a right to his concerns. At some point the decision might become a joint one. But his inability to even listen to Sandy's plan not only deprived her of the chance to think out loud but also made her less likely to consider his feelings in the final decision.

Whether it's money, the kids, or mothers-in-law, there are unsafe subjects in every family. A woman doesn't talk to her Catholic relatives about having an abortion. The same woman might not risk telling her husband that she might be able to sleep better if they got separate beds if she was afraid he'd be too offended even to entertain the possibility. He might not tell her about a problem he's having at work if he was afraid she'd respond with unwanted advice. He might not want to burden her with financial worries (or share the decision making). It's not necessarily a question of keeping secrets, though most family members have a few. Rather, it's just hard to tell the people you live with everything. With friends, few subjects are off limits.

In conversations between friends, little misunderstandings can be passed over or forgotten between breaks in contact. Disagreements between people who live together are harder to forget.

The relationship between friends is voluntary; you can leave if you want to, and therefore it's safer to be honest. You can talk over painful or embarrassing subjects, reveal self-doubts, try out different sides of yourself, and be who you are.

People show caring and respect by the quality of their listening.

Friends who listen make us feel interesting, and their interest inspires us to say more interesting things. Their receptivity is transformative: by listening intently to us, our friends make us larger, more alive. That's the glory of friendship.

A Good Friend Is a Good Listener

When you want to talk to a friend, do you begin by asking how he or she is doing before getting to what's on your mind? This common courtesy often results in perfunctory listening. You've asked, you've listened; now it's your turn.

Most people think more about what they want to say than about what is being said to them. To be a good friend, learn to listen better. Once in a while, try approaching a friend with the intention of finding out what's on his or her mind and listening for an extended period of time.

A friend is someone with whom you can talk about almost anything. With such friends we take turns as selfobjects, willing for a time to submerge ourselves and be there without strings for our friend. Friendship grows with mutual disclosure. So do we. The compassion friends offer when they listen to our triumphs and worries deepens us; their understanding keeps us from feeling alone—and helps us understand ourselves.

Friendship deepens us; it also broadens us. Friendships expand our definition of ourselves and awaken unrealized possibilities, possibilities that aren't part of the scripted roles we play in our families. With many friends we can express many sides of ourselves. The intimacy of friendship, the selfobject function, strengthens us. Mutuality, the sharing function, stretches us.

"I Wish I Had More Friends."

Write down the five most important things on your agenda for the next seven days.

Was spending time with a friend on the list? Was trying to strike up a friendship with someone at work or the gym on the list? Was strengthening an already established friendship by expressing your affection on the list?

With friends we are easy, but, sadly, it isn't easy to find time for friendship. When I asked people what interfered most with talking to friends, by far the most common response was "I'm too busy." In crowded and hurried lives, greedy obligations squeeze out anything optional, like spending time with friends. But even though many of us are preoccupied these days, it's more than lack of time that undermines friendships.

When Friends Take Sides

After her divorce Maggie turned to her friends. They saw her through the shock of separation and the months that followed. Though she felt adrift, at least she wasn't alone.

Maggie's friend Liz was also divorced and disillusioned; she understood what it was to be single again, having to start all over, the indignities and misunderstandings. The two women had known each other for nine years, ever since they met at a workshop (ever since, in fact, they both skipped the afternoon session and ran into each other at a local art gallery).

Liz made friends easily. She embraced Maggie with her warmth and held her with her intelligence and keen eye for the pretentious and foolish. They met often for lunch or for a drink after work, enjoying conversations about their jobs, families, friends, what they were reading, how they felt—if any subject was off limits, they hadn't come to it yet.

Maggie met Dominic three years after her divorce. As chance would have it, he lived in Liz's building, and on several occasions she ran into him in the downstairs lobby. She found him attractive but couldn't imagine speaking to him; he seemed so unapproachable. It came as a surprise, therefore, when he started talking to her one Saturday afternoon and, after no more than five minutes, asked her out. To her equal surprise, she found herself accepting.

If opposites attract, they were a perfect match. Maggie had the ruddy complexion and emotional reserve of her Scottish ancestors, while Dominic was Greek, with dark hair and olive skin and an openly expressive nature. She liked the way his mind worked, all intuition and confidence. What a relief after all those pale, shadow men her friends had fixed her up with!

The passion Maggie felt with Dominic was thrilling. Unfortunately, as she soon found out, the price to be paid was a series of equally passionate quarrels. Dominic was jealous of her time, her friends, and just about everything else. Though he might sometimes be busy for days, he expected her to be available whenever he wanted to see her. When she wasn't, there were storms of jealousy.

When Maggie told her friends about all the trouble she was having with Dominic, they were sympathetic. Liz got angry. She considered Dominic's possessive jealousy abusive and thought Maggie was wrong to put up with it. "I'd never let a man treat *me* that way," she said.

After one particularly violent outburst, Maggie decided not to see Dominic for a while. As long as they'd been going together, Liz had held back the worst of her criticism, but now that Maggie was considering ending the relationship, Liz spoke up. Maggie would be better off without him, she said. In this opinion, Liz was not alone. All of Maggie's friends felt the same way: if Dominic was causing her so much unhappiness, she should dump him.

Unfortunately, sympathy can get in the way of empathy. Unable to suspend their own emotional impulse, which was to rescue Maggie from the grief she shared with them, her friends urged her to put an end to what was making her so unhappy. That's what friends often do when we complain about someone: they take our side and push us to retaliate.

It's one thing to honor a friend's right to happiness, but far more difficult to respect her right to put up with unhappiness if she decides to go to war for love.

Maggie was buoyed by the sympathy of her friends but felt pressured by their urging her to break up with Dominic. While it's comforting to have someone to share your feelings with, it's not always comforting to be told what to do about them.

After a while Maggie stopped talking to her friends about Dominic. She wasn't only angry at Dominic; she also loved him. While it's okay for us to criticize our own loved ones, it's a mistake for friends to agree. Our griping expresses one side of our ambivalence—and leaves us free to do whatever we decide about the relationship. But a friend's agreeing that someone we're close to is a terrible person is a boundary violation.

There is no formula for an empathic response, but it may help to remember that there are two sides to every conflict. Understanding—

empathy—therefore often means acknowledging uncertainty. If a person hasn't acted to resolve a problem, there's probably a reason.

Liz might have said something like "You sound pretty unhappy, but I guess you're not sure what to do." Instead she said, "Dominic's not good enough for you. If you go back to him now, you'll hate yourself for it."

• • •

There are things that have no place in friendship, and judgment is one of them.

• • •

Showing empathy to friends doesn't mean just caring about them; it means listening to their point of view, whether or not you agree with it. Friendship doesn't require neutrality or total acceptance; but before they disagree or give advice, real friends listen.

Here is an example of a friend struggling to be empathic from Paul Auster's novel *Leviathan*. Peter's friend Sachs is telling him about the accident in which he fell off a four-story fire escape, trying to explain that he feels responsible because he wouldn't have been out there if he hadn't been flirting with a woman.

> There were questions I wanted to ask him then, but I didn't interrupt. Sachs was having trouble getting the story out, talking in a trance of hesitations and awkward silences, and I was afraid that a sudden word from me would throw him off course. To be honest, I didn't quite understand what he was trying to say. There was no question that the fall had been a ghastly experience, but I was confused by how much effort he put into describing the small events that had preceded it. The business with Maria struck me as trivial, of no genuine importance, a trite comedy of manners not worth talking about. In Sachs's mind, however, there was a direct connection. The one thing had caused the other, which meant that he didn't see the fall as an accident or a piece of bad luck so much as some grotesque form of punishment. I wanted to tell him that he was wrong, that he was being overly hard on himself—but I didn't. I just sat there and listened to him as he went on analyzing his own behavior.[1]

It's said that men and women bring different expectations to friendship, that women have a basic commitment to attachment, men to independence. Thus it may be difficult for men to listen to themes of depen-

---

[1] Paul Auster, *Leviathan* (New York: Viking, 1992).

dence and attachment, while women may have trouble accepting a friend's choice to go her own way. This may be true in general, but relationships don't exist "in general." Relationships take place between individuals. While those individuals may have been brought up to have certain expectations, the fate of our relationships doesn't depend on conditioned traits of character, but on how we choose to act toward one another.

To be with other people authentically—that is, to respond to them as they are, not as we want them to be—is no easy feat. This ability depends on an awareness of ourselves as self-contained individuals who relate by listening to and accepting other separate and autonomous individuals.

Maggie and Liz's attachment was built on shared interests. When Maggie began to feel differently, the friendship waned. The two friends didn't know how to tolerate the differences that were emerging between them. Maggie felt she was betraying Liz whenever she was happy. Neither of them knew how to talk about the feelings they were experiencing. Liz felt abandoned by Maggie. Their differences and their inability to talk about them formed a widening gulf. As in so many situations where differences between friends can't be talked about, the friends drifted apart.

When Maggie eventually worked things out with Dominic, she stopped seeing Liz altogether. Years later she would say to someone offhandedly, "Oh, we just lost touch."

Resolving Conflicts with Friends

Why, if Maggie was able to work things out with her jealous and demanding boyfriend, wasn't she able to resolve the conflict with her like-minded and appreciative friend? Here's the irony of listening in friendship:

The same elective quality of relationship that enables friends to speak freely about so many subjects makes them less likely to speak openly about problems between them.

The binding nature of family ties makes it more urgent to speak up about our unhappiness in those relationships. While friends do sometimes voice complaints to each other, they are less likely to talk about serious problems between them, like envy, jealousy, or resentment. Because the ties of friendship aren't as obligatory as those of family, there's a greater fear that friends will abandon us if we voice complaints to them. Sadly, when such feelings are strong, friends often drift apart.

• • •

**If you have a gripe about someone and the relationship
is optional, let it go. But if you have a grievance about
someone you care about, find a way to say something.**

• • •

People who hesitate to speak when something is bothering them
often imagine that those brave souls who do simply have more confidence
in themselves. Perhaps. But most of the people I've known to tell friends
that something is bothering them were just as worried about saying so as
those who keep silent. What enabled them to take the risk wasn't only
respect for themselves and their right to their feelings, but also respect for
the relationship—and for their friends.

The longer you avoid telling a friend that something's bothering
you—say, that you wish your friend wouldn't make a habit of bringing
along a third person when you get together—the more preoccupied you
become with your grievance. In your internal debate about whether or
not to complain, you probably imagine phrasing your complaint in such
a convincing way that your friend will have to hear you. In fact, the most
effective way to address an impasse between friends is to take into account
what you imagine your friend's position to be.

• • •

**Acknowledging your friend's position releases
him or her from brooding about it and opens him
or her to hearing your side.**

• • •

Let's say that you always seem to be the one to call a certain friend
about getting together. You're not the sort of person to keep score, but her
never inviting you to do anything together troubles you. You're starting
to wonder if she really likes you. You hesitate to say anything because she
might feel attacked. What to do? Tell her all of that. Use your ability to
empathize to anticipate how your friend might feel about what you have
to say. "Something's been bothering me, but I've hesitated to bring it up
because I didn't want you to think I was blaming you. Actually, this may
have to do with my own insecurity ... "

• • •

Sometimes an honest complaint can save a friendship.

• • •

Michelle got tired of Arlene's constant complaining—about her jerk of a boss, her numerous aches and pains, and her rich repertory of boyfriend troubles. But she didn't want to say anything. She didn't want to hurt Arlene's feelings. (Isn't that what we tell ourselves when we don't want someone to get mad at us?) So instead of saying anything, she just stopped being available when Arlene called, and the friendship withered and died.

When friends don't speak up about what's bothering them, grievances gnaw at the relationship. Even if it doesn't completely resolve the conflict, hearing each other's position makes a big difference. The best place to start to address an impasse between friends is not to state your position but to consider what your friend might be feeling and try to acknowledge that in a way that invites him or her to elaborate.

Few friendships last long if all one person does is complain about things. We all have troubles in mind, but remember that listening, especially to complaints, is a burden. If you have a friend who takes advantage of your willingness to listen without reciprocating, you can accept this burden until you get fed up—like collecting enough frequent-flyer miles to trade in for the right to walk out on the friendship. Or you can say something.

A running friend of mine used to complain about all the trouble he was having with his stepson. I'd listen sympathetically and occasionally offer advice (it's okay, I have a license). But if my friend talked for more than a few minutes, he'd get self-conscious (maybe partly *because* I have a license) and apologize. I'd remind him that in our relationship complaining was a two-way street. I didn't mind hearing about his problems because I was grateful for the time he spent listening to mine.

When two people are locked in silent grievance, the best way to open the subject is to ask about the other person's feelings. This applies especially to mutual misunderstandings. Don't be too quick to tell your side. In cases of major misunderstanding, concentrate first on listening to the other person. Save your feelings for later. But if your friend has hurt you and doesn't know it, eventually saying something about how you feel may be the only way to keep your resentment from poisoning the relationship.

Alice and her husband were both independent and regularly did things like go out to dinner or to the movies separately. Alice's friend Marie, on the other hand, didn't feel comfortable socializing without her husband.

So the two friends sometimes got together alone, but more often they did things as couples, as Marie preferred. They both understood their different situations, but each came to feel that she was doing more of the accommodating. Gradually, they saw less and less of each other.

Marie was hurt. She was disappointed that Alice wasn't more sympathetic to her situation. The less they saw of each other, the more Marie brooded over how hurt she felt; and the more she brooded, the more she imagined confronting Alice. Could Alice's feelings conceivably mirror her own? It was a possibility she hadn't considered, but she decided to take a risk in the interest of preserving the friendship.

Marie called and said she imagined Alice must be frustrated by her having trouble getting together except as couples. Alice, relieved to have her feelings acknowledged, said yes that was true, but deep down she worried that Marie didn't really like her enough to want to do things alone together.

Once Marie had broken the ice by showing concern for Alice's feelings, the two friends were able to talk about their misunderstanding and resentment—feelings that often seem too threatening to talk about. The basic conflict didn't disappear—Alice still preferred to get together alone with Marie, and Marie still had trouble going out without her husband—but it no longer festered. The two friends now understood each other, and their friendship endured.

How to Offer Constructive Criticism to a Friend

There are times when just listening to a friend you feel is making a mistake is less than honest. However, if you feel like offering advice, it's a good idea to first ask if your friend wants to hear it.

"Would you like to hear a suggestion about this?"

"Are you interested in a second opinion?"

"Have you definitely decided to ... ?"

Advice implies criticism, and even well-intended criticism can backfire. You may have been trying to be honest or simply have been thoughtless; either way your criticism may make your friend feel attacked. If you suggest that a friend change something he or she isn't interested in changing (or likely to change), your comments, however well-meaning, can leave the friend feeling resentful.

Sometimes when we give our opinion, we feel rejected if our friend doesn't follow it.

"Why did you ask for my advice if you weren't going to take it?"

Taking advice means considering it, not necessarily following it. The best kind of advice has no strings attached. A good listener allows friends to accept or reject suggestions without acting slighted.

See how your friend responds to your initial comments before going on. Don't become so attached to convincing a friend of the rightness of your assessment—of *her* decisions—that you are insensitive to her right to decide what to do. If your friend seems defensive about your advice, pull back and let her talk.

• • •

**The time to press your point of view is
when you disagree with a friend about what
you should do, not the other way around.**

• • •

If you're not sure how your friend feels about your advice, ask.

"What do you think?"

"Do you want me to say more about this or not?"

"Should I go on, or have you pretty much made up your mind?"

Do Friends Outgrow Each Other or Just Forget
How to Listen?

For all too many people the story of friendships is a history of broken connections. The loss of friends may not be as wrenching as those of people who live together and share destinies, but the process is similar. We make friends in one set of circumstances—in college, say, or starting a new job or, like Maggie and Liz, as veterans of divorce. Then one or both of us changes; we move on, and the connection becomes harder to sustain.

The reasons we marry at twenty aren't the same reasons we stay married at thirty or sixty, but friends, who have fewer ties to bind them, are less likely to do the maintenance it takes to sustain a relationship through major life changes. A lot of that work involves respecting each other's differences and learning to listen when it doesn't come easily.

Gil and Roy were friends in high school. Both were basketball players and good students, and they gravitated together naturally. It was a friendship based on shared interests and the kind of wisecracking teenage boys use to test themselves. Their listening to each other, if you can call it that, took the form of taking turns showing off.

As they grew older, Gil found Roy's constant ribbing exasperating but often invigorating, too. Others just found it annoying. Once, when they were in their thirties, they were at a basketball game and Roy had had a few beers. It was just after the great Kareem Abdul-Jabbar had changed his name from Lew Alcindor, and for some reason he became the target of Roy's abrasive humor. Every time Jabbar missed a shot, Roy would holler, "Hey *Lew*, nice shot, *Lew!*" He was really starting to bother the people around them, but Gil didn't say anything. After the game a couple of guys confronted Roy, called him an asshole and knocked his glasses off. Later, when Gil teased him about the incident, Roy got very upset, and the two friends stopped speaking to each other.

A couple of years later Roy called Gil, and the friendship was renewed, only now it seemed more superficial, at least to Gil. Roy still seemed so adolescent. He was always posturing, looking for an angle, a spin, a take.

Together the two friends attended their twentieth high school reunion. Gil remembered how the waves of emotion and memory washed over him but that Roy remained his old wisecracking self. Afterward the two of them went out for a drink with Gil's old girlfriend.

Janice, who was still sensationally pretty, brought out the old competitive edge between the two friends, who spent an hour in the bar tossing barbed comments back and forth. Gil didn't think Janice was very impressed by their performance, and later he felt a little embarrassed.

Much later Gil learned that Roy had taken Janice home that night and the two of them had had an affair. The way he found out was that Roy called him, all upset, to tell him that Janice had broken off with him. Gil was furious. It seemed like such a devious and hostile thing for Roy to have done—not just to score a conquest with his old girlfriend, but to keep it secret. Why, if there was nothing sneaky in what Roy had done, hadn't he said anything about it? Still, when Roy turned to Gil to nurse him through his hurt, Gil was forgiving, the way friends are.

The next time the two friends got together was when Gil invited Roy to his annual company picnic. Roy, who'd again had a few beers, started making jokes about private things Gil had said to him about various members of the company. Gil was embarrassed and tried to shut Roy up but wasn't very successful. The following week, Gil wrote a letter to Roy saying that he didn't trust him anymore, that he didn't plan to see him again, and that he didn't want Roy to contact him.

Gil (who would later outgrow and shed his first marriage) found this act—deliberately severing a tie that had become a burden—quite liberating. It felt like a declaration of self-respect. Thinking about the end of the friendship, he remembered Woody Allen saying that the things that mean the most in this world, the things that are the most enjoyable, come naturally. You can't work at them.

That's how we sometimes feel, but that doesn't make it so. Maybe when we're kids friendship comes easily, but as we get older we may have to work at it. Working at making friends and keeping them may go against the grain, but that's true of a lot of things worth doing. Gil's friendship with Roy may have become one of those relationships that persist out of habit even though they are fundamentally unrewarding. But many friendships, even based on a more solid connection, may require repair from time to time. For friendships to grow with you, you may have to put in some effort.

One important ingredient in getting the listening you deserve is cultivating relationships based on mutual exchange. This means remaining open enough to form new relationships and selective enough to drop those that aren't worth the effort. Deepening relationships requires a balance between self-disclosure and listening. But then, inevitably, many of us find ourselves stuck in relationships with people who have trouble listening. Instead of remaining bitter or fatalistic, it's possible to teach them to listen—by setting an example and, if necessary, asking for reciprocation.

Having friends means making time for them. If friends come second, if you're too busy working to be with your friends, what are you working for? Keeping friends means being willing to work at it. Not all the time certainly, but listening sometimes when it's hard and speaking up sometimes when it's necessary.

For friendship to flourish the relationship must be given priority. That means finding time for each other, and it means making a real effort to listen to each other. At work, however, there are more important things than relationships. Aren't there?

Getting Your Point of View Across at the Office

Marshall and Steve were thoroughly charming to Marianne when she applied for a job at the small publishing firm where they were respectively publisher and senior editor. They asked the usual questions about her training and experience but spent more time talking about what a great place it was to work. Marianne needed little convincing. Any small publisher, she felt, would be better than the huge conglomerates where editors were drowning in profit-and-loss statements and books of substance were considered with suspicion and irony.

Marianne felt she could learn a lot from Marshall and Steve. She knew she had the makings of a good editor, but her experience at the large firm where she'd been a valued assistant hadn't prepared her to negotiate contracts or conduct other such business matters with ease.

Marianne was thrilled when she received a letter offering her the job a week after her interview. She'd worked a long time for this moment, and she finally had what she wanted.

Marianne was surprised at how quickly her responsibilities built up. Who would have thought that so many of the bright young authors she was attracting to the firm (and some older ones as well) would need so much hand-holding?

Marshall and Steve seemed happy to have Marianne around. But she soon discovered that they considered themselves chiefs and her an Indian. They were friendly enough, in a superficial way, but they never thought to really include her. Between meetings and appointments they would talk to each other and not to her. They'd discuss people she didn't know and exchange inside jokes. Their constant showing off, meant to entertain and impress, made her feel that all they wanted from her was an audience.

When Marianne discovered that they went out to lunch together every Wednesday without inviting her, she felt a humiliating shock of alienation. Later she learned that the firm's small board of directors had forced them to hire a woman editor and that Marshall and Steve resented this intrusion into what they considered their fiefdom.

Another reason Marianne felt shut out was that Marshall and Steve were such great friends. So close were they that people invariably referred to them as Marshall-and-Steve, as though they were inseparably a pair, a single hyphenated unit. People invited Marshall-and-Steve to parties, the booksellers asked Marshall-and-Steve to serve on committees, and authors and agents referred to Marshall-and-Steve as the savviest and most devoted people in the business. The fact that they were both so popular with authors, literary agents, and other industry people only underscored Marianne's sense of isolation.

One reason they were so well liked was that they were so accessible. They loved publishing, they loved books, and they loved the way their authors looked up to them with the total, trusting eagerness that people whose identities are invested in their writing reserve for those who appreciate their work. So Marianne was perplexed by their response when she approached them about the manuscripts she was having problems with. Marshall and Steve made a pretense of listening, their brows furrowed in concern like state-funded bureaucrats on autopilot, but they asked no questions. When she was done, they told her just to continue to do her own good work.

These encounters left Marianne not just disappointed but humiliated. But instead of getting angry, she felt ashamed of asking for help. She didn't really need much help; what she wanted was simply some support. More than advice, she needed collegiality, that comforting sense of shared enterprise that had sustained her through the hard years of school and publishing apprenticeship.

Shut out socially, then judged inadequate just because she'd asked for feedback, Marianne became cold and hostile. Not wanting to give her antagonists the satisfaction of exposing her real feelings of rejection, she took refuge in contempt and punished them with silence.

The atmosphere in the office became so unpleasant that Marianne thought about quitting. But she was a single mother and didn't have that luxury.

It was at this point that Marianne started dating a publishing executive at another firm, a tall man with gray eyes and a large spirit. Quinn was a man of patient sweetness, but he too was divorced, and at first he and

Marianne were somewhat tentative with each other. Then love took over and work became less important.

The trouble was, as Marianne now began to see, that from the beginning she'd expected a lot from Marshall and Steve. When she'd interviewed for the job she mistook their friendliness for an offer of friendship, and when that promise wasn't fulfilled, she became bitter. Then, too, she wanted both to be appreciated as competent and given the guidance she needed as a beginner. That these motives are somewhat contradictory doesn't make them unreasonable. Marianne's bitterness was due partly to the frustration of her own inflated expectations and partly to her colleagues being too caught up in their own lives to be open to a new person.

Things changed at work when Marianne stopped worrying so much about Marshall and Steve. Now that her personal life was full, she was less interested in their friendship or even their approval. And now that she felt better about herself, she was no longer willing to put up with blatant unfairness.

When Marshall, who was filling out the annual review, rated her "mediocre," Marianne refused to sign it. "I want to talk about this," she told him evenly. When Marshall said he didn't have time, she insisted. "You *have to* talk to me. Make time." He sighed theatrically but agreed.

"You *know* I deserve a good evaluation," Marianne told him when they finally met. "What's the problem?"

"I call it as I see it," Marshall said, getting up to leave.

"Please sit down," Marianne said. "We have to talk about this."

And talk they did. Marianne acknowledged that she may have expected too much when she arrived, but she also pointed out that she'd been treated like a second-class citizen and she was tired of it. They didn't have to be friends, she said, but they did have to get along. She spoke with dignity, but also with intensity.

When Marianne finished saying what was on her mind, Marshall apologized. He changed the evaluation, and after that both he and Steve started treating her with more respect. In return, Marianne dropped her belligerent attitude, but she was no longer willing to put up with not being listened to.

Why were Marianne's bosses so unresponsive for so long, and why now all of a sudden did they start to listen to her? Could it really be that all she had to do was speak up?

Marshall and Steve had allowed their resentment about being pressured to hire a woman to turn into a grudge. Unwilling to confront *their* bosses, they took out their frustration on Marianne, shutting her out and treating her as someone to be seen but not heard. What they didn't realize was that grudges have no place at the office.

• • •

Holding on to resentment of people you have to work with punishes you as much as it does them.

• • •

It may be a cliché, but people who work together are a team, and sometimes it's necessary to get past personal feelings that interfere with the functioning of the group.

Although Marianne had tried to complain, her expectations got in the way. Like many of us, she wanted to be liked, and hoped to be friends. That's fine if it happens, but Marianne had allowed her wish to be friends to take priority over doing her job and insisting on being treated fairly. It's harder to confront your boss if you need him or her to like you than it is if you just want respect.

Anxious and uncertain about speaking up—lest Marshall and Steve not like her—Marianne spoke to them in a nervous, tentative way. At the other extreme, speaking up in a shrill voice doesn't get you much respect either. No one coached Marianne on exactly what to say or how to say it, but the assurance she drew from her relationship with Quinn resulted in her lowering the pitch of her voice and speaking more directly. She didn't just want to air her feelings; she wanted things to change.

On Secretary's Day, Marshall and Steve gave the receptionist a dozen carnations with a card signed from the two of them. Marianne was furious. They responded by saying that this was a social gesture and they could do what they liked. She told them that this was an office, not a social setting, and that she wouldn't be excluded like this. The next day they apologized.

Keep in mind the difference between dissent and defiance as a response to being treated unfairly. *Defiance* means disagreeing to attack the other person's position. *Dissent* means disagreeing to stand up for what you believe. It's the difference between saying "You're wrong" and "This is what I think."

Defiance is reactive, a counterphobic response to the temptation to deference. A dissenting opinion is much easier to hear than a defiant one.

Marianne now realized that she was entitled to be listened to, and when important issues arose, she insisted on it. Knowing she could fight back effectively made her more relaxed, and so there was less often a need for it. No longer anxious for Marshall and Steve's approval, as though she were a child and they parents, Marianne lost her dependence, her need to please: she was an independent person. The company, as usual, published some very good books that year, and an author Marianne had brought in had a great success, both critical and commercial. She and Marshall and Steve had a wonderful celebration with him one evening, and their gratification was genuine and shared.

Marianne's unhappy experience at the office is instructive for two reasons. First, her colleagues' lack of consideration illustrates one of the greatest mistakes senior people make in work settings: not listening to their subordinates. Second, that insensitivity placed Marianne in the kind of situation that tempts us to feel like victims, wearing our suffering as a rebuke to the villains we hold responsible. The fact that Marianne was a woman suffering at the hands of two men also permits those who care to see this as an example of men as tyrants and women as martyrs. Let's look at these issues one at a time.

A Good Manager Is a Good Listener

Managers are expected to lead the people under them. Unfortunately, people get promoted because they were good at the jobs they were doing, not because they've proven themselves as managers. In fact, according to the Peter Principle, people tend to advance until they reach their level of incompetence. As a result, many managers pay more attention to the product than to the people producing it—to the detriment of both.

"Yes, Master."

The more powerful and admired the boss, the more people tend to hold back their opinions rather than risk angering the person in charge.[2] Good

---

[2] That's one reason presidents make a mess of things: they fail to correct misguided poli-

managers make it safe for everyone to offer their ideas and opinions—even ideas that appear to be wrong or at odds with their own beliefs. This openness accomplishes two things: it adds to the pool of information, which makes for more informed decisions, and it makes people feel included in the decision-making process. The larger the pool of ideas, the better the final decision is likely to turn out. And the more people feel they have participated in the decision making, the more willingly they are likely to act on the decisions that get made.

Effective managers are proactive listeners. They don't wait for members of their staff to come to them; they make an active effort to find out what people think and feel by asking them.

The manager who meets frequently with staff members stays informed and, even more important, communicates interest in the people themselves.

An open-door policy allows access, but it doesn't substitute for an active effort to reach out and listen to people. The manager who doesn't ask questions communicates that he or she doesn't care. And if he or she doesn't listen, the message is "I'm not there for you." Even if a manager decides not to follow a subordinate's suggestion or not to give someone a raise, listening with sincere interest conveys respect and makes the employee feel appreciated.

When Marshall and Steve hired Marianne, they were impressed by her maturity. They thought of her as a self-sufficient person who would share the load. You might think that as experienced people they would have been more sensitive to a new colleague's need for support. But the truth is, they did their best work outside the office. When they sat down to court an agent or an author, they were very sensitive.

Marshall and Steve didn't offer Marianne any supervision because *they* never got any. What didn't occur to them was that their friendship had sustained their own need for support. The mistake they made in dealing with Marianne was thinking about her only as a worker and not as a person. Interest in peers may come easily; but, even if it doesn't come

---

cies because their advisors trip over themselves to agree with the boss. If agreement equals access, bad choices are unlikely to be challenged (cf. the wars in Vietnam and Iraq).

naturally, senior people must take an interest in junior people. They're the ones who get the work done.

• • •

Communicating by memo or e-mail doesn't substitute for personal contact, because it closes off the chance to listen.

• • •

Simply going through the motions of meeting with people doesn't work. The fake listener doesn't fool anyone. Poor eye contact, shuffling feet, busy hands, and disingenuous replies, like "That's interesting" and "Is that right?" give them away. The insincere supervisor's lack of interest in the conversation betrays a larger problem: lack of interest in the person.

Failure to listen isn't necessarily a product of meanness or insensitivity. Anxiety, preoccupation, and pressure can undermine the skills of even a good listener. The point is, really, that at work, as in every other arena of life, listening requires a little effort.

Effective managers develop a routine in which communication time is an integral part. They meet with their staff and ask questions. They don't react before gathering all the facts. If they don't know what their people are thinking and feeling, they ask—and they listen.

Listening to Empower

A family therapy institute invited six leaders in the field to serve as a board of advisors. At their initial meeting each of the first five experts made suggestions about how the institute could improve their programs. The sixth member of the board took an entirely different approach. He asked everyone on the staff to talk about what they most wanted to accomplish and how they thought he could support them in that. It was a remarkably productive way to bring out the best of people's ideas.

What If Your Boss Doesn't Listen?

If at this point we were to leave the subject of listening at the workplace, we would have fallen into the easy habit of reducing a complex subject to a simple formula: thoughtful managers listen to what their employees have to say. Where does that leave those who don't get listened to?

When we don't feel heard by our superiors, few of us give up right away. We write memos, we ask to meet with them, we try to communicate our needs and convey our point of view. Then we give up. Eventually we do what Marianne did: complain to other people.

Once Marianne came to the conclusion that her colleagues were uninterested and unavailable, she started griping to the receptionist.

Gossip is a form of consciousness lowering. The rules of the game are simple: players are free to run down anybody who's not in the room. (Hint: If you play this game, don't leave the room.)

Triangulation—ventilating feelings of frustration to third parties rather than addressing conflicts at their source—takes on epidemic proportions in work settings. Letting off steam by complaining about other people is a perfectly human thing to do. The problem is that habitual complaining about superiors locks us into passivity and resentment. We may have given up trying to get through to the sons of bitches, but by God we don't mind saying what we think of them—as long as they aren't within earshot.

I once worked in a clinic with six other therapists, where everyone except the director went out to lunch together every day. Guess what the main topic of conversation was? The director and what a rigid guy he was. And guess what the group did about it? Complained regularly among themselves, as though they were a resistible force and he were an immovable object.[3]

But, some of you might be thinking, my boss *really is* insensitive! I've *tried* to talk to him; he just doesn't listen!

I don't doubt it. People aren't promoted because they're good listeners. They get promoted because they're good workers, or maybe good talkers. Moreover, positions of authority encourage the directive side of human nature, often at the expense of receptivity. The mistake people make in trying to get through to unreceptive superiors is the same mistake most of

---

[3]When I became the director of an outpatient psychiatry department, I remembered this lesson. I scheduled weekly staff meetings, the first half of which was devoted to discussing patients, and the second half was for the staff to bring up anything they were unhappy about, any suggestions they had, or anything they could think of that would make their jobs more rewarding. The result was a pretty cohesive unit.

us make in dealing with the difficult people in our lives: We try to change them. And when that doesn't work, we give up.

• • •

You don't improve relationships by trying to change other people, but by changing yourself in relation to them.

• • •

Start by examining your expectations. What do you want, and how do you expect to go about getting it? Are you, as Marianne was, expecting to have your personal needs met at the office? Do you work hard and wait patiently for the boss to tell you that you're doing a great job, like a good little boy or girl? Have you learned to seek a reaction by being clever rather than competent or by being pleasing rather than productive?

The workplace isn't a family. Yet many of us relate to our bosses as though they were our parents. The alternative is to think of yourselves as two self-respecting adults who happen to occupy different positions at the office. Marianne wanted Marshall and Steve to take her seriously, but she hadn't taken herself seriously. Trying too hard to be liked and waiting patiently for the boss to recognize your worth are examples of not taking yourself seriously.

The chairman of the department of psychiatry once complained to me that certain faculty members responded to him as though he were their father. I had to laugh.

One of the things that comes with a position of responsibility is becoming the object of people's attitudes toward authority. (I think it's called transference.) Supervisors should remember this when they meet with their subordinates. When employees are summoned to meet with the boss, they may expect a reprimand—why else would the boss call you in?—rather than an open forum. Supervisors must break through this anxiety by asking questions that show interest. And listening to the answers.

Listening within Limits

Leslie was sympathetic when her secretary told her about the problems she was having at home. But once Donna discovered what a willing listener Leslie was, she started taking up more and more time talking about her problems. Donna's troubles were beginning to interfere with work getting done, and Leslie was getting annoyed. She wanted to be understanding, but she didn't want to be Donna's mother. What to do?

If you have a good relationship with someone at work and that person has a personal problem, your willingness to listen helps lighten the burden. But some people are so full of their problems that they take advantage of anyone willing to listen.

When personal conversations start keeping you from your work, cut them off gently but firmly.

> "I'd like to hear more, but I have to get back to work."

> "This all sounds pretty painful. I hope you have somebody to talk to about these things?"

> "Sorry, I think I hear my mother calling."

Listening is important at work because it enables people to understand each other, get along, and get the job done. *But:* Don't get too personal. Don't let your compassion (or desire to be appreciated) allow someone's talking about his or her personal problems to interfere with work. This may be happening if you're the only person he talks to or if she uses your sympathy as more than an occasional excuse for not getting things accomplished. A good supervisor keeps channels of (business) communication open—and keeps them focused on the task at hand—by asking for frequent feedback about how things are going (at work).

> "What do you like and dislike so far about working here?"

> "Is there anything you think we should change to make things smoother?"

> "How do you feel about ... ?"

> "What's your reaction to ... ?"

Remember that it can be intimidating for subordinates to give criticism or make suggestions. If you want them to feel safe enough to open up, reassure them that you appreciate their ideas.

"I'm glad you spoke up."

"Thanks for letting me know ... "

"I didn't realize ... I'm glad you told me."

Listening to the people you work with isn't the same as becoming friends with them. Many people worry that if they allow themselves to get personal at the office, things might get sticky. But those who think that effective teamwork isn't about listening (it's about getting things done) are wrong. Without being heard we are diminished, as workers and as people.

Exercises

1. In your next conversation with a friend, note any tendency to drift away while the other person is talking. How much effort would it take to concentrate on listening for exactly two more minutes? How much effort is this friendship worth?

2. Make a list of friends you'd like to be closer to. Then note things you know those people like to do. Pick a friend and try to arrange doing that activity together.

3. Become a proactive listener. If you are a supervisor, manager, teacher, therapist, parent, or otherwise in a position of authority, find a time in the coming week to ask a subordinate what ideas or feelings about your mutual enterprise he or she might have but has not had a chance to tell you about. Be sure to make that person feel appreciated for opening up to you. If the person says nothing, say that's fine; if anything comes to mind later, you'd be glad to hear about it.

4. Think of a difficult colleague or supervisor. How do your interactions with that person usually go? What do you do? For the next time you meet with that person, plan to concentrate on listening and drawing out his or her point of view. Afterward, evaluate your listening and its impact on the relationship.

Epilogue

An epilogue is where the author can be expected to wax philosophical. Here, for example, I might tell you that better listening not only transforms personal and professional relationships (which it does) but can also bring understanding across the gender gap, the racial divide, between rich and poor, and even among nations. All that may be true, but if I'm going to indulge in the unearned right to preach, maybe I should confine myself to matters closer to home. After all, I'm a psychologist, not a philosopher.

Having read this far, you've probably been reminded of some things you already knew but perhaps also come to see that listening is even more important and difficult than people realize. The urge to be heard is so compelling that even when we do listen, it's usually not with the intent to understand but to reply. And, as if that didn't make listening hard enough, at times of heat and conflict it takes a real effort to overcome, or at least restrain, the reactive emotionalism that jolts us into anxiety and out of sympathy with each other.

Few things can do as much to bring mutual understanding to your relationships as responsive listening—hearing and acknowledging other people's thoughts and feelings before voicing your own. You can make responsive listening a habit but, like any new habit, it takes practice.

One of my least favorite remarks has come from certain individuals in therapy to improve their relationships. They've complained. I've listened sympathetically. Then I've suggested things they could do to start giving and getting the understanding they say they long for. Then comes The Comment: "Why does everything have to be so artificial? Why can't we just talk to each other?" I hate that! They *were* talking, and it wasn't working.

It's annoying when people say that it's unnatural to hold their response until they've acknowledged what the other person has to say, because this protest seems so stubborn and self-defeating. But the thing that really annoys me about this comment is that it's true: good listening *doesn't* come naturally.

Listening is a skill, and like any skill it must be developed. But although listening can be looked at this way—as a performance—it can also be looked at another way, as a natural outgrowth of caring and concern for people.

*   *   *

Caring about people doesn't require a lot of thought; it's something you feel. Caring about others almost automatically impels you to act with consideration for them. This consideration isn't wholly unselfish, because caring about someone means that your well-being is tied up with theirs. When a bad thing happens to someone you love, something bad happens to you as well. But *showing* that you care, suspending your own interests and making yourself receptive, isn't always easy.

Listening a little harder—extending what we do automatically, extending ourselves a little more—is one of the best ways we can be good to each other. Attending a little harder to other people—enough to hear their feelings, enough to consider their point of view—this takes a little effort.

Caring enough to listen doesn't mean going around selflessly available to everyone you encounter. Rather, it means being alert to those situations in which someone you care about needs to be listened to.

*   *   *

Ironically, our ability to listen is often worst with the people closest to us. Conflict, habit, and the pressure of emotions makes us listen least well where listening is most needed. As we move outside the family circle to those we care about but don't live with, we tend to be more open, more receptive, and more flexible. It's not—as we're sometimes accused of— that we care more about our friends than about our family but that these relationships are less burdened with conflict and resentment.

You won't get far with your efforts to listen better without running into the problem of your own emotionality. Listening better requires not only a greater openness to others but also a greater awareness of yourself. Do you express yourself in a way that makes listeners anxious and defensive? If so, what can you do about it? (If the answer is nothing, then that's the improvement you can expect in the listening you get.) Under what circumstances do you become reactive and give advice or interrupt or make jokes instead of listening?

*   *   *

Concern for other people is an instinctive expression of the best part of us. Unfortunately, frustrations at home and a sense of powerlessness in the wider world mean that we don't always act with generosity and concern.

*   *   *

Everywhere around us we're encouraged to claim our victimhood and right to bitterness. This feeling of injured entitlement can be understood as a product of insufficient emotional nourishment. People who are hungry for attention are suffered, shunned, or shamed. Others let them know in some way that their need to be heard is excessive. And where does that leave them? Hungry for attention. And so the problem of listening, like all human problems, is circular: inadequate appreciation makes us insecure in ourselves and less open to others. The listening we don't get is the listening we don't pass on.

Our inability to get the attention we crave leaves us feeling powerless—a feeling reinforced by living in a world marked by economic decline, crime, pollution, and bureaucratic ineptitude. So it's not surprising that we've lost faith in our capacity to make a difference. Public disillusion and private disappointment deplete and discourage us. We feel put upon and let down, and so, naturally, we turn our resentment outward and our sympathy inward.

When you feel beleaguered and insecure, it's natural to think about looking out for number one. Unfortunately, self-absorption is self-defeating. Trapped in self-consciousness, we become polarized and resentful. Sadly, anger and despair have fueled a decline in concern and a retreat to the dead end of preoccupation with ourselves.

You can't simply reverse the process of misunderstanding, but you can realize that relationship problems are circular, and circular patterns can be broken—if someone is willing to make the first move.

The great reward of making that move is that listening allows us to be open, generous, and connected; to touch others' lives and to enrich them and us in the process. Listening—empathic listening—promotes growth in the listener, the one listened to, and the relationship between them.

That better listening enhances our own well-being is the natural perspective of psychology, in which all human behavior is seen as motivated by the agendas of the self. But when you narrow down human relations to a collection of selves, and the self to the early conditioning of the child, what you have left is fixed characters, and you're stuck with them.

It's a dogma of American life that all actions are motivated by self-interest. But this dogma is false. The tendency to view our lives on the planet from the perspective of individualism obscures the larger view that we are part of systems within systems: the family, the extended family, the community, the nation—vast networks of associations. The truth is that looking inside ourselves can show us only part of the reason for feeling empty and unfulfilled.

Should the idea of self-interest include interest in others? Yes. Benevolent self-interest goes hand in hand with interest in others. But is it only a matter of enlightened self-interest to take an interest in other people?

Trade-offs have their place in the conduct of life. But it would leave too much out of the story of human affairs to give an account of relatedness to others only in terms of utilitarianism.

Caring about other people, which takes shape in political justice, the relief of suffering, and the love of family and friends, is fundamental to our sense of who we are and what makes our lives hang together. Pressures that block or obscure this impulse reduce, even damage us.

Respect for human dignity doesn't mean only feeling sympathy for others or doing for them. It means respecting them enough to listen to them, to hear and appreciate their voices—to view them as subjects, worthy of hearing, not just as objects of our needs.

Listening to others is an ethical good, part of what it means to have just and fair dealings with other people. Listening is part of our moral commitment to each other.

*   *   *

Listening better to those you're closest to is easier when you remember that we are separate selves. Openness and autonomy are correlated. If you are to have the courage to be yourself, to stand squarely on your own two feet, then you must accept that other people are entitled to their own point of view. The idea isn't to separate yourself from others but to let them be themselves while you continue to be yourself.

Learning to listen involves a paradox of self-control: controlling yourself and letting go of control over the relationship. It's like letting someone else drive. To listen, you have to let go.

Trying harder to understand another person's perspective takes effort, but it isn't just a skill to be studied and practiced. Hearing someone is an expression of caring enough to listen.

One of the things I've hoped to do in this book is to help restore a sense of balance to the way we think about relationships. First because seeing our relationships as mutually defined enables us to change what we get out of them by changing what we put into them. And second because recognizing that we live in a web of relationships, which give meaning and fullness to our lives, may inspire us to a little more generosity and concern for other people.

Does talk of rebalancing relationships and rediscovering concern sound a little pious? After all, you probably picked up this book to learn a little more about listening, not to read a sermon on benevolence. Sorry. But maybe the sympathy for other people that we're born with is something we have to remind ourselves to express from time to time.

We all believe in fairness and respect for the rights of others. We believe in compassion and justice and that everyone has a right to be heard. Of course these standards are regularly violated. It remains that they are valid standards. And they do from time to time galvanize us to action—as when we somehow manage to listen instead of arguing in the midst of a heated discussion or when we remember to take a little extra time to hear what's going on in someone's life.

The obligation to listen can be experienced as a burden, and we all sometimes feel it that way. But it is quite a different thing to be moved by a sense that the people in our lives are eminently *worth* listening to, a sense of their dignity and value. One thing we can all add a little more of is understanding—respect, compassion, and fairness, the fundamental values conveyed by listening.

*   *   *

As I said at the beginning of this book, the reason we long so much to be listened to is that we never outgrow the need to communicate what it's like to live in our separate, private worlds of experience. Unfortunately, there is no parallel need to listen. Maybe that's why listening sometimes seems in short supply. Listening isn't a need we have; it's a gift we give.

Index

309

About the Author

Michael P. Nichols, PhD, Professor of Psychology at the College of William and Mary, is the author of *Stop Arguing with Your Kids*, among numerous other books. He is a well-known therapist and a popular speaker.